VIGOR:

HOW TO ELIMINATE SUGAR IN FOOD

Discover How to Overcome Sugar
Addiction & Detox Your Body
by Eating Delicious Alternative Food
With a Tasty 21 Meal Plan Full of Healthy,
Sugar-Free Recipes

Written by:
ALICE FLOUR

ALICE FLOUR

© Copyright 2021 - All rights reserved.

The content contained within this book may not be reproduced, duplicated or transmitted without direct written permission from the author or the publisher.

Under no circumstances will any blame or legal responsibility be held against the publisher, or author, for any damages, reparation, or monetary loss due to the information contained within this book. Either directly or indirectly.

Legal Notice:

This book is copyright protected. This book is only for personal use. You cannot amend, distribute, sell, use, quote or paraphrase any part, or the content within this book, without the consent of the author or publisher.

Disclaimer Notice:

Please note the information contained within this document is for educational and entertainment purposes only. All effort has been executed to present accurate, up to date, and reliable, complete information. No warranties of any kind are declared or implied. Readers acknowledge that the author is not engaging in the rendering of legal, financial, medical or professional advice. The content within this book has been derived from various sources. Please consult a licensed professional before attempting any techniques outlined in this book.

By reading this document, the reader agrees that under no circumstances is the author responsible for any losses, direct or indirect, which are incurred as a result of the use of information contained within this document, including, but not limited to, errors, omissions, or inaccuracies.

Table of Contents

INTRODUCTION 10

CHAPTER 1: WHAT IS SUGAR? 12

    DISCOVER THE ROLE OF SUGAR: 12
    BEFORE SUGAR: SWEETNESS..... 12
    MOVING TO OUR DAYS: THE SUGAR ERA 13

CHAPTER 2: A GUIDE TO NATURAL SWEETENERS 14

    COCONUT SUGAR 14
    DATE SUGAR 14
    RAW HONEY 14
    MAPLE SYRUP 15
    MAPLE SUGAR 15
    POWDERED HONEY 15
    MOLASSES 16
    STEVIA 16
    XYLITOL 16

CHAPTER 3: HOW TO BREAK FREE OF YOUR SUGAR HABIT 18

    CUT OUT LIQUID SUGARS 19
    CHOOSE FRESH FRUITS 19
    ALWAYS COMPARE FOOD LABELS 19
    EXTRACTS FOR FLAVOR 20
    NON-NUTRITIVE SWEETENERS 20
    SUBSTITUTE OR REPLACE IT 20
    BENEFITS OF GOING SUGAR-FREE 20

CHAPTER 4: WHY IS IT BAD TO TAKE SUGAR? 22

    IMMEDIATE EFFECTS 22
    "ADDED SUGARS" AND "SUGAR FREE" 23
    FINAL THOUGHTS: DEFEAT YOUR BAD HABITS 23
    YOU CAN START TRYING TO MAKE SOME OF THE FOLLOWINGS YOURS: 23

CHAPTER 5: BREAKFAST AND SNACKS 26

    1.   CHEESY LOW-CARB OMELET 26
    2.   APPLE & CINNAMON PANCAKE 26
    3.   CREAM CHEESE PANCAKES. 27
    4.   BULGUR PORRIDGE 27
    5.   RHUBARB MUFFINS 28
    6.   TURKEY-BROCCOLI BRUNCH CASSEROLE 28
    7.   GUACAMOLE TURKEY BURGERS 29
    8.   HAM AND GOAT CHEESE OMELET 29
    9.   BREAKFAST SMOOTHIE ... 30
    10. BAGELS 30
    11. BUCKWHEAT AND GRAPEFRUIT PORRIDGE 31
    12. EGG AND VEGGIE MUFFINS 31
    13. QUINOA CONGEE WITH CAULIFLOWER 32
    14. WINTER FRUIT SALAD 32
    15. BUCKWHEAT GRANOLA .. 33
    16. MUSHROOM FRITTATA 33
    17. BREAKFAST CREPES 34
    18. CHERRY BERRY BULGUR BOWL 34
    19. CITRUS BLUEBERRY MUFFINS 35
    20. PINEAPPLE BREAD 35
    21. ZUCCHINI BREAD 36

22. Keto Scrambled Eggs 36
23. Strawberry & Spinach Smoothie 37
24. Tomato and Zucchini Sauté 37
25. Banana Matcha Breakfast Smoothie 38
26. Tofu and Vegetable Scramble 38
27. Basil and Tomato Baked Eggs 39
28. Berry Breakfast Bark 39
29. Chia and Coconut Pudding 40
30. Apple Filled Swedish Pancake 40
31. Apple Topped French Toast 41
32. Bacon & Egg Muffins .42
33. Cauliflower Breakfast Hash 42
34. Vegetable Frittata 43
35. Vegetable Omelet......43
36. Mexican Style Burritos. 44
37. Fast Microwave Egg Scramble 44
38. Bacon & Eggs 44
39. Summer Veggie Omelet.. 45
40. Sweet Pancakes........... 45
41. Summer Breakfast Parfait 46
42. Cauliflower Potato Mash 46
43. Garlic Bread 47
44. Fried Egg 47
45. Quick Breakfast Yogurt Sundae 47
46. Coconut Breakfast Porridge 48
47. Whole-Grain Pancakes 48
48. Granola With Fruits .49
49. Egg Muffins 49
50. Immunity Booster Smoothie 50

CHAPTER 6: FIRST COURSES 52

51. Healthier Egg Salad Sandwich 52
52. Sunday's Sausage Sandwich 52
53. Mexican Style Tortillas With Pork 53
54. Veggie Pasta Primavera 54
55. Meat Pasties 55
56. Stuffed Portobello Mushrooms 55
57. Grilled Halibut With Veggies 56
58. Burgoo 57
59. Mexican Beef Stew..... 58
60. Italian Veggie Soup... 58
61. Korean Beef Soup 59
62. Bell Pepper Stew 59
63. She-Crab Soup 60
64. Sweet Potato and Pumpkin Soup With Peanuts 60
65. Spicy Chicken Stew 61
66. Tomato-Based Stew ... 61
67. Down South Corn Soup. 62
68. Carrot Soup 63
69. Bean Field Stew 63
70. Pasta Salad 64
71. Chicken, Strawberry, and Avocado Salad............. 64
72. Lemon-Thyme Eggs.... 65
73. Spinach Salad with Bacon 65
74. Dijon Roasted Brussels Sprouts 65
75. Quinoa Stuffing......... 66
76. Italian Rice Bites 66
77. Southwestern Sweet Bake 67

78. Rice Pilaf 67
79. Warm German Potato Salad 68
80. Roasted Cauliflower with Apple and Dill 68
81. Vegetarian Baked Beans 69
82. Jicama and Veggie Salad 69
83. Broccoli Cheese Casserole 70
84. Italian Bean & Broccoli Sauté 70
85. Roasted Roots & Fruits with Creamy Balsamic Drizzle 71
86. Cherry Tomatoes On The Side 72
87. Ham And Asparagus Rolls With Cheese 72
88. Creamy Cheddar Sauce With Ham And Sherry 72
89. Crispy Potato Pancakes 73
90. Scalloped Potatoes With Leeks And Country Ham 73
91. Basic Cream Sauce 74
92. Parmesan-Crusted Asparagus 74
93. Southern Cheese Grits 75
94. Italian Ricotta-Chestnut Fritters................ 75
95. Home Fries 76
96. Quinoa, Corn, And Bean Salad 76
97. Beet And Goat Cheese Salad 77
98. Cauli-Slaw 77
99. Tabbouleh 78
100. Mint Cabbage Salad 78

CHAPTER 7: SECOND COURSES WITH SIDE DISH . 80

101. Peppered Broccoli Chicken 80
102. Buttery Cod 80
103. Lime Baked Salmon 81
104. Turkey Coriander Dish 81
105. Flank Steak Beef ... 82
106. Sage Beef 82
107. Roasted Tomato Brussels Sprouts 82
108. Simple Sautéed Greens 83
109. Garlicky Mushrooms 83
110. Green Beans In Oven 83
111. Parmesan Broiled Flounder 84
112. Wild Rice Salad With Cranberries And Almonds .. 84
113. Low Fat Roasties 85
114. Roasted Parsnips 85
115. Beef, Olives, And Tomatoes 86
116. Easy Lime Lamb Cutlets 86
117. Sumptuous Lamb And Pomegranate Salad 87
118. Pork Spare Ribs 88
119. Lime Trout And Shallots 88
120. Fish And Salsa 88
121. Crab Legs 89
122. Teriyaki Chicken And Broccoli 89
123. Coconut Lime Chicken 90
124. Roasted Vegetable And Chicken Salad 91
125. Chicken Satay 91

126. CHICKEN FAJITAS WITH AVOCADOS 92
127. CRISPY BUTTERMILK FRIED CHICKEN 92
128. GARLICKY CHICKEN WITH CREAMER POTATOES 93
129. HONEY LEMON GARLIC CHICKEN 94
130. BAKED LEMON PEPPER CHICKEN DRUMSTICKS 94
131. PORK CHOPS WITH GRAPE SAUCE 95
132. ROASTED PORK & APPLES 95
133. PORK WITH CRANBERRY RELISH 96
134. SHRIMP & VEGGIES CURRY 96
135. LEMON AND HONEY PORK TENDERLOIN 97
136. DIJON PORK TENDERLOIN 98
137. AIR FRYER PORK SATAY. 98
138. PORK BURGERS WITH RED CABBAGE SLAW 99
139. BALSAMIC-GLAZED CHICKEN 99
140. CAJUN SALMON 100
141. TROUT AND ZUCCHINIS 101
142. BBQ PORK RIBS 101
143. GLAZED PORK SHOULDER 102
144. LAMB ROAST 102
145. PORK CHOPS IN PEACH GLAZE 102
146. SPICY CHICKEN DRUMSTICKS 103
147. BEEF AND CHORIZO BURGER 104
148. PEPPERED CHICKEN BREAST WITH BASIL 104
149. HOMEMADE HAMBURGERS 105
150. CHICKEN MEATBALLS ... 105

CHAPTER 8: DESSERTS 108

151. FLOURLESS CHOCOLATE CAKE 108
152. PEANUT BUTTER CUPS 108
153. ICE CREAM BROWNIE CAKE 109
154. FRUIT PIZZA 109
155. CHOCO PEPPERMINT CAKE 109
156. ROASTED MANGO ... 110
157. FIGS WITH HONEY & YOGURT 110
158. RASPBERRY CAKE WITH WHITE CHOCOLATE SAUCE ... 110
159. BERRY ALMOND PARFAIT 111
160. CAPPUCCINO CUPCAKES 112
161. PUMPKIN SPICED ALMONDS 112
162. PUMPKIN CUSTARD . 113
163. STRAWBERRY SHAKE 113
164. CINNAMON PROTEIN BARS 114
165. CHOCÓ COOKIES..... 114
166. CHOCOLATE AVOCADO ICE CREAM 114
167. CHEESE CRISP CRACKERS........................ 115
168. COCONUT MILK SHAKES 115
169. LAVA CAKE 116
170. CHEESE CAKE 116
171. CAKE WITH WHIPPED CREAM ICING........................ 117
172. WALNUT-FRUIT CAKE 118
173. DARK CHOCOLATE CAKE 118
174. STRAWBERRY & WATERMELON POPS 119

175. BAKED APPLES WITH DRIED FRUIT 119
176. RASPBERRY ALMOND TART 120
177. OATMEAL BUTTERSCOTCH COOKIES 120
178. AVOCADO MOUSSE .. 121
179. CINNAMON TOASTED ALMONDS 121
180. CINNAMON APPLE CHIPS 121
181. DARK CHOCOLATE ALMOND YOGURT CUPS 122
182. TOMATO & CHEESE IN LETTUCE PACKETS 122
183. MANGO MOUSSE 122
184. BANANA SPLIT SUNDAE. 123
185. TZATZIKI DIP WITH CAULIFLOWER 123
186. RUSTIC PEAR PIE WITH NUTS 124
187. RASPBERRY PEACH COBBLER 125
188. APRICOT SOUFFLÉ ... 125
189. CINNAMON APPLE POPCORN 126
190. BLACKBERRY CROSTATA 126
191. CHIA AND RASPBERRY PUDDING 127
192. PALM TREES HOLDER 127
193. ALMOND CHEESECAKE BITES 128
194. STRAWBERRY MOUSSE.... 128
195. BLUEBERRY LEMON "CUP" CAKES 129
196. BAKED MAPLE CUSTARD 129
197. ALMOND FLOUR CRACKERS 130
198. CREAM CHEESE POUND CAKE 130
199. OATMEAL PEANUT BUTTER BARS 130
200. PEACH CUSTARD TART... 131

21-DAY FOOD PLAN 134

CONCLUSION 136

Introduction

The term "sugar-free" is often used to describe foods such as cookies, gum, and drinks, that have chemical and artificial sweeteners in place of sugar. Artificial sweeteners approved by the U.S. Food and Drug Administration include saccharin, acesulfame potassium, aspartame, neotame, and sucralose. These artificial sweeteners are found in products like Sweet 'N Low, Equal, and Splenda. These products are indeed free of refined white sugar and are often calorie-free, but simply being "sugar-free" does not mean they are healthy. Diets heavy in foods with artificial sweeteners are as unhealthy as diets high in refined white sugar.

Research shows that similarly to sugar, artificial sweeteners desensitize the body's reaction to sweet food, leaving the body unsatisfied. This results in consuming food in excess to satisfy hunger. Artificial sweeteners are much sweeter than regular sugar, causing a person's proverbial "sweet tooth" to be continuously overstimulated. Over time, that overstimulation changes tastes and preferences. Naturally sweet foods such as fruit don't taste as good as they once did, and non-sweet, simple foods such as vegetables can become truly unappetizing.

Studies also show that artificial sweeteners are just as addictive as white sugar. A 2007 study at the University of Bordeaux in France found that rats overwhelmingly preferred saccharine to cocaine, suggesting the addictive quality of the substance. Researchers provided rats with a choice of saccharin-sweetened water and intravenous cocaine. The rats could press a lever and receive either a shot of cocaine or a sip of saccharin-sweetened water as often as they wanted. The animals chose the high from artificial sugar water 94 percent of the time. Researchers in the study believe their findings reveal that the concentrated sweetness of artificial sugars creates a more intense pleasurable sensation and addiction than cocaine does.

CHAPTER 1:

What is sugar?

Discover the role of sugar: in modern day food habits, how and why its consumption is inflated and a series of simple steps that will make you feel better by embracing a healthy way of eating and thinking about food. But before going forward, let's dive back in the time when sugar didn't even exist yet. Let's learn the origins of sugar and how this substance acquired the popularity and success that we are used to.

Before sugar: sweetness

We could say that people always loved sweet, tasted food, in both Europe and the rest of the world, honey, dates, and other sweet foods were very appreciated and commonly used as sweeteners. Ancient history of Mediterranean left us writings and other reliable proofs of this.

Honey is the oldest known sweetener, some unique 12,000-year-old cave paintings in Spain show women collecting honey. At the time, women used the honey for culinary purpose, just as we do today, but also for making mead and for cleaning wounds.

Sugar was imported in Europe in the late 10th century, and its usage was reserved to the upper classes, who used it mostly as a sweetener and as a drug for about five more centenaries.

In 1099 the Europeans, when they conquered Jerusalem with their Crusades, learnt the secrets on how to produce sugar. At the time it was certainly a big discover, embracing a chance to grow a new ingredient and to unexpectedly start to run one of the biggest businesses of all time.

During 15th century, the Spanish start importing sugar and setting up plantations which led them to increase slavery to run their new business. Shortly after Columbus discovered America, the Spanish started exporting sugar plantation to grow their profit, and then Pedro Cabral of Portugal lands on a shore which was discovered to be Brazil to establish even more plantations of sugar, with new mills and more sophisticated methods.

From 16th to 18th century, sugar got an extremely powerful boost around the globe, though it was primarily a spice for the rich people that really caught on thanks to the imports of coffee, tea, and chocolate, which are today certainly known to fully combine with sugar.

Since second half of 19th century, after first and second industrial revolutions occurred, sugar became more and was already popular all around the world, so much that the world's biggest and most advanced sugar refinery was built in Williamsburg at that time.

The biggest sugar company and brands were founded during 20th century, a controversial centennial for our spice: doctors from the American Medical Association's Council on Food and Nutrition suggested for the first time that a "limit in consumption of sugar would have been healthy for the people", who were at this point already consuming tons of the so-loved sweet spice.

Moving to our days: the sugar era

Today, most of the packaged food that we normally buy and eat contains added sugar.

Since it has been discovered, sugar has been the Prime ingredient to exalt, alone, the flavor of other food, making his own history for many centuries. If one didn't know anything about the story of sugar, it would be comprehensible to list it as one main if not the most important ingredient for recipes of actual confectionery and sweets, but it is not just like that.

Sugar in our times has been used more and more often by industries to "secretly" exalt the flavor of packaged food.

Of course, it is reliable to check the list of ingredients printed on the back of food packages to acknowledge that (or if) they contain any sugar, but it is very common to find out that most of the food we buy contains at least a little bit of sugar or other sweeteners.

Food industry knows very well the properties of sugar and uses them at their best. In fact, there's a formula that industries use to obtain the perfect quantity of sugar to be added to the food they produce to make them sweeter than they would normally be and that makes us want to eat more of that food: this is called the "happiness point".

Neuroscience helps to understand this phenomenon: the complex molecules of sugar divide in simpler ones during digestion progress, and what reaches our brain is the activation of "the ways of the dopamine" through these molecules. Dopamine is a neurotransmitter, strongly involved in the feeling of satisfaction for human beings. It is therefore warranted that if we eat any food containing the quantity of sugar which makes it reach the "happiness point", it will give us a satisfying feeling that will make us want to eat more of that specific aliment.

CHAPTER 2:

A Guide to Natural Sweeteners

Naturally sweetened recipes such as those found in this book are free of refined white sugar and artificial sweeteners. Natural, whole-food sweeteners including honey, coconut sugar, pure maple syrup, and molasses are used instead.

Please be mindful that although these natural sweeteners promote health and are full of vitamins and minerals, they should be used in moderation and with knowledge of how each sweetener affects the body.

Coconut Sugar

Coconut sugar, often called coconut palm sugar, is made from the flowers of the coconut tree. Coconut sugar does not have the same tropical flavor usually associated with coconuts. It closely resembles brown sugar in appearance and taste and has a distinctly sweet scent. It caramelizes like sugar, so it works particularly well in baking. Coconut sugar replaces sugar cup-for-cup in recipes. It's naturally full of vitamins and minerals like potassium, amino acids, magnesium, zinc, and iron. Coconut sugar is a whole food and does not drastically impact blood sugar levels. It's a safe diabetic sugar substitute, with a low glycemic index of 35.

Date Sugar

Date sugar is dehydrated, ground-up dates. Dates are a healthy fruit high in vitamins, fiber, and minerals, and they provide delicious natural sweetness to a recipe. Dehydrating and grinding the dates to sugar does not compromise the health benefits of whole dates as the dry product is a convenient natural sweetener. Because date sugar is dehydrated, it can drain baked goods of moisture, so most recipes with date sugar need a lot of liquid. Date sugar is a pure fruit, so it has a relatively high glycemic index and is not a good choice for diabetics.

Raw Honey

Raw honey is unfiltered, unprocessed, and straight from the beehive. It's an alkaline food and contains the vitamins, enzymes, minerals, and water needed to sustain life. Raw honey contains vitamin C, amino acids, B vitamins, and minerals such as calcium, magnesium, zinc, phosphate, and potassium. When a recipe calls for honey, any kind of honey will do. However, to get all of the antibacterial, anti-inflammatory, and antiallergic health benefits, raw honey is recommended.

Raw honey can aid in neutralizing toxins in the body, has cancer-fighting properties, can help reduce fevers, and can soothe coughs and sore throats. It is often used topically to help heal acne, skin rashes, or eczema. When raw honey is mixed with cinnamon or ginger, it can help calm constipation, upset stomachs, and nausea.

Processed honey, which is any honey that does not specifically say it's raw, is void of most of the health benefits mentioned. Processing occurs to create a product that is clear and lighter in color than its natural state, which most consumers prefer. It also keeps it from crystallizing as quickly as raw honey does. Antibiotics and added sweeteners such as high-fructose corn syrup and water are often present in processed honey.

All honey is processed similarly to refined sugar in the body, so honey is not a low-glycemic food, ranking a 50 on the glycemic index scale. It should be used with care by those who suffer from diabetes.

Maple Syrup

Pure maple syrup is produced by boiling the sap of the maple tree. It contains amino acids, magnesium, zinc, and other vitamins and minerals. It has become popular in the health food industry because it is a natural source of antioxidants, similar to broccoli and blueberries. Antioxidants have been proven to fight cancer cells and decrease the effects of aging. Maple syrup is a natural source of energy and nutrition when eaten raw. It's a healthy sweetener, but should be consumed sparingly for those with diabetes, as it ranks 54 on the glycemic index.

Maple syrup comes in different grades, from extra light to dark. In the United States, there are two grades of maple syrup, Grade A and Grade B. Grade A typically has a milder flavor and pale color. Grade B has a very sharp maple flavor and is darker in appearance. Both grades of maple syrup work equally well for cooking and baking.

Maple Sugar

Like maple syrup, maple sugar also comes from the sap of the maple tree. The maple tree sap is boiled until no water remains, creating a solid maple sugar product. Solid maple sugar is sold as a bar or ground into a granulated powder and sold by the bag. It is almost twice as sweet as refined sugar and has a distinct maple flavor. Maple sugar holds up well in baked items and caramelizes well.

Different brands of maple sugar have different size maple sugar granules. If one brand is too coarse, you can process the sugar in a blender to create a finer powder.

Powdered Honey

Powdered honey is dehydrated honey. It can be called honey powder, granulated honey, or dried honey. There are many different brands of powdered honey available, and the quality can vary greatly. Differences in products include whether or not the honey is organic, whether it is pure or contains fillers, and how finely it is powdered. Some products have thicker, bigger "grains" while others are extremely fine and look like golden baking soda.

Honey powder is a great natural sweetener with some but not all of the health benefits of raw honey. It contains many vitamins and minerals and has a lower glycemic index than white sugar. It also has a subtle floral flavor and provides a great texture to baked goods, keeping the final product moist and tender.

Molasses

There are a few different sources of molasses, but the two most common in the United States come from the sugar cane plant and the sorghum plant. Molasses is a great alternative to sugar because of its slightly sweet taste, its high mineral and vitamin content, and its accessibility. There are a few varieties of molasses that can come from the sugar cane plant, with blackstrap molasses ranking as the most nutritious option. Blackstrap molasses contains high levels of iron, calcium, potassium, copper, and magnesium, which are all important nutrients for the body. Sorghum molasses also has significant nutritional benefits and is a natural source of sweetness. Sorghum molasses (also commonly called sorghum syrup) is an unprocessed product that contains many important minerals and B vitamins. Whichever type of molasses is used, organic, unsulphured molasses is recommended. Blackstrap molasses ranks 55 on the glycemic index, with sorghum ranking at 50.

Stevia

Stevia is a sweet herb native to South America and has been used for centuries. It's almost 300 times sweeter than sugar and is most commonly used in a liquid or powder form. It makes a great sweetener for teas and drinks.

Stevia is a healthy food, but there are many products on the market today that contain stevia with additional unhealthy fillers such as chemicals, animal byproducts, and sugar. Stevia is a plant that is so sweet that it is impossible to make a product in which it replaces sugar cup-for-cup. For instance, one would never use one cup of stevia to replace one cup of sugar in a recipe because pure stevia is too concentrated. If a stevia product claims it is equal to sugar in use, it contains unhealthy fillers to create the extra bulk. Look for plain stevia, either in liquid or powder form, with just one or two ingredients listed on the label.

Xylitol

Xylitol is a natural sugar alcohol found in the fiber of plants and fruit. It is commonly extracted from certain types of tree bark, cornhusks, and mushrooms. It is a sugar substitute with almost a third of the calorie content of sugar. Xylitol has a flavor and consistency similar to sugar and therefore is ideal for a variety of recipes. However, it does not caramelize like sugar when baked, so this sweetener works especially well in ice creams, drinks, or frostings.

People are often familiar with xylitol because of its association with sugar-free gum and candy. Although other unhealthy ingredients are sometimes associated with sugar-free products like those, xylitol is a whole food, is nontoxic, and is very safe for consumption. It is important to note that because xylitol is a sugar alcohol, high consumption can upset the stomach or cause bloating. Introduce this sweetener into your diet slowly and monitor your body's reaction to it closely so it is not eaten in excess. Xylitol, like stevia, is acceptable for the candida diet. Not only is it acceptable, but it is the only sweetener that actually fights candida and helps kill yeast growth and infections. Xylitol doesn't raise blood sugar levels and can even promote dental health as it has been proven to help fight plaque and rebuild tooth enamel. Xylitol is unsafe for pets, and pregnant women should only use xylitol after consulting with their doctor.

CHAPTER 3:

How to Break Free of Your Sugar Habit

So, maybe you're at risk of diabetes, or maybe you already have it but don't know what you can do to lessen your sugar consumption habits. The good news is that it isn't that bad to break these habits. It can take a while, and you need willpower, but if you have that, you should be able to fight off the habits as well. All you have to do is to be willing to make some significant changes to your diet. Ultimately, people are hardwired to desire sugar. When we didn't have easy access to sugar, we needed to want as many carbs as possible to keep ourselves healthy and alive; the carbs would help us to create fats and would also help to keep us full. However, nowadays, because we don't have to forage or hunt and gather for food, we have our own problems. Currently, the problem is that food is too easy to find. Because it is so readily available, you run into the problem of potentially storing up too much fat as a direct result. However, you can learn to prevent this from being a problem.

We are hardwired to want to go for those sugary choices the same way most animals are. Studies have shown that animals will go out of their way to choose sugar over cocaine in lab tests. However, sugar is not good for us in excess, as we have established thus far. This means that you will need to be mindful of what you are doing to prevent yourself from getting ill. You will need to figure out how you can make sure that you do not unintentionally poison yourself with too much sugar. Now, let's look at what goes into breaking that habit—or even that addiction, in some cases.

Before we begin, consider the fact that sugar comes in all sorts of forms. It comes in the form of sucrose and fructose. Lactose and maltose are two others. Sucrose can be found, as well. As you can see, hover, they all end in "-ose." That is the sign that you are looking at a sugar if you don't see the actual word written in front of you. Because sugars come in so many different forms, it can be difficult to truly eliminate them. It can be impossible for you to figure out what you will need to do to prevent yourself from getting ill from these effects. You will need to make sure that you are working hard to ensure that your diet is well-managed. Ultimately, if you are able to recognize these different forms of sugar, you will be able to prevent yourself from eating things that aren't going to help you.

As an additional note, consider the fact that you don't need to cut out all forms of sugar—you just want to cut it out when it is added to your diet. This means that it is okay to eat whole food that breaks down into carbs, but you don't want to eat something that is laden with high fructose corn syrup. Eating foods that are loaded up with sugars can be a huge problem, and most people don't even realize that they are doing it, they just do so because they think that since the word sugar isn't on the ingredient list, they are safe to eat it without a concern.

If you are ready to cut out sugar from your diet, there are a few steps that you should follow to help yourself do so. These aren't necessarily difficult to do, but many people find that it is hard to stick to them. They get caught up in the cravings, or they give into the withdrawals that they feel when they do cut them out. Your body gets used to those higher levels of sugar in your diet and comes to rely on them; when you cut them out, you are likely to run into some symptoms as your body has to develop and adjust to its new normal.

Cutting sugar by tossing out added sugar sources is the first step to making sure that you can eliminate sugar. You must take the time to genuinely cut it out in the first place if you have added sugar options in your home, such as white and brown sugars, or also eliminating the honey. If you are going to make yourself coffee or tea, you want to make sure that you aren't adding these. At first, make sure that you do so gradually. You want to start out by cutting the amounts of sugar in half and slowly weaning down over the period of a couple of weeks. This is what is best for you.

Cut out Liquid Sugars

All too often, people drink sugars that they don't even realize. Soda is one of the biggest sources of sugar that we get. Additionally, you can see that adding honey or sugar to coffees and teas is another common source, as is drinking juice. None of these are very healthy options; you need to make sure that you are cutting out those sugars over time. Coffee and tea are fine, so long as you are mindful of the sugars that you put into them.

Choose Fresh Fruits

If you want something sweet, go for fruit, but still, be mindful. Fresh fruit is usually the best for you, but you can also go for unsweetened frozen fruit or even canned fruit if it is in water or natural juices. Make sure that you avoid the fruit that is canned in heavy syrups; this is a common source of sugars that people don't realize that they are using. You can also use fruit as a natural sweetener. If you are going to use a sweetener of some sort for yogurt, cereals, or oatmeal, this is a great option for you. Fruit is a great option to flavor your teas or water as well if you are someone that's used to sweetened and flavored drinks.

Always Compare Food Labels

When you look at your food labels, make sure that you choose those that have the lowest amounts of added sugars. Many foods are naturally going to have carbohydrates in them—and that's okay in moderation. You must make sure that you are cutting out those high added sugar foods to keep yourself healthy. This means that if you have a food with 22 grams of sugar and 18 are added, and you can also choose a food that has 25 grams of sugar with just 4 or 5 added, the second food is going to be the healthier choice because it doesn't involve adding any natural sugars.

Extracts for Flavor

Instead of relying on sweeteners like sugar, you can use extracts like vanilla or lemon to add some richness and flavor without the calories.

Non-Nutritive Sweeteners

If you just can't cut the sugar entirely, you can make it a point to limit the sugar that you do consume, switching it out with non-nutritive sweeteners. However, treat this as a crutch rather than a permanent option. It is better for you to just keep things natural and avoid adding any sweeteners entirely.

Substitute or Replace It

If you are cooking something, there are several options that you can use as a way of avoiding the sugar entirely. You could use spices to enhance the foods instead of using sweeteners. You can also use ingredients such as applesauce to replace sugar and fats in many baking dishes as a nice way to cut out the added sugars.

Benefits of Going Sugar-Free

The results of eliminating sugar and artificial sweeteners can be astonishing, and the long- and short-term benefits can be wide-ranging. Physical benefits go beyond just weight loss. By allowing more room in the diet for healthy foods, vital nutrients can promote increased energy, a stronger immune system, improved complexion, better digestion, steadier blood sugar levels, and improved sleep. In addition, long-term health risks of developing heart disease, diabetes, obesity, and diseases associated with these conditions can be reduced, if not eliminated.

Eliminating or even reducing processed sugar and artificial sweeteners from your diet has the added benefit of promoting improved mental health. You may experience clearer thinking, decreased irritability, fewer mood swings, and an increase in self-control. Less mental energy directed toward fighting cravings or addictions promotes better overall health.

CHAPTER 4:

Why is it bad to take sugar?

Try to imagine, for a second, the gear of a beautiful watch with all its small pieces carefully assembled by a master watchmaker of the highest quality: if we poured a jar of honey on it in a very short time the whole mechanism would jam, because it would be literally stuck in every component of the sugar contained in honey. This is metaphorically what happens scientifically in our bodies when we let it absorb excess sugar over time. Counting the sugar we add to every coffee, tea, the sugar in sweets, and even the large number of refined grains we tend to eat in excess such as pizza, bread, pasta, potatoes, sandwiches, sauces, salty snacks... we are used to eating too much sugar for our bodies.

Immediate effects

A large amount of sugar that is metabolized and absorbed quickly causes a sudden increase in blood sugar in our body, which reacts with an equally rapid overproduction of insulin.

Medium-term effects and increased risk of developing diseases

If repeated continuously over time, this phenomenon is not well tolerated: the mechanism tends to become saturated, leading to an increased risk of developing insulin resistance, i.e., decreased insulin effectiveness. Overweight, obesity, and the general inflammatory state of the body are related.

Long-term effects and chronic diseases

Development of chronic diseases such as diabetes, metabolic syndrome and some types of cancer.

There are also side effects of excessive sugar intake, such as skin damage.

In fact, excess sugar facilitates the creation of a bond with proteins in the body, resulting in structural alteration and loss of function of these proteins.

This process is called glycation, and a very simple example is what happens on people's skin: sugar binds in particular to collagen and elastin, two proteins contained in skin tissue, causing accelerated aging. Skin aging is a visible manifestation of the damage that sugar creates, but what happens to collagen and elastin also happens in all other tissues, even those not visible. The number of sugars must necessarily be reduced also because of the implications it has with childhood obesity and in adulthood with cancer and diabetes: undoubtedly those who eat too much sugar are more likely to get sick. However sugars are not always easily identifiable and knowing how to read labels is fundamental in order to choose foods with low sugar content and to individuate the hidden ones.

"Added sugars" and "sugar free"

According to the legislation on food claims, a product can be defined on the label "low sugar content" if it contains no more than 5g of sugars per 100g for solids or 2.5g of sugars per 100 ml for liquids.

The term "sugar free" refers to a food with no more than 0.5 g of sugars per 100 g or 100 ml, while the wording "without added sugars" concerns food in which no sugar has been added and any other indication that may have the same meaning for the consumer. It is allowed to be used on labels only if the product does not contain added mono- or di-saccharides or any other food product used for its sweetening properties.

If the food naturally contains sugars, the following indication must appear on the label: "naturally contains sugars".

Final thoughts: defeat your bad habits

Sugar has become part of our life in a way that we did not choose and did not control at all. Even though it has become a strong habit for our body and for our lifestyle, it is not at all impossible to get rid of these problems. After listing all the "bad sides" of sugar to open your eyes about its long story from the past to today's industry leading to its popularity, and naming all its possible, more sustainable substitutes, it is now time to show you the way to really protect yourself, that is to forcefully exercise a series of linked decisions and carry them out for long enough to make them become new, good habits.

You can start trying to make some of the followings yours:

1. **Distinguish your home** from the rest of the environments that are frequented, avoid buying and keeping certain types of food at home: the house must become a kind of "Temple of Health" where certain things do not fit.

2. **Decide that sweet things become exceptions** to be savored with taste only on special occasions and that these should be limited to once a week.

3. **Decide to eliminate the use of unnecessary added sugar** such as that in coffee, juice, soda, alcohol.

4. Try to **"replace" instead of "eliminate"** altogether, for example, the less healthy sweets with fruit, or use stevia (or any other from the list above) as a natural sweetener and decide that the daily dessert is given by a couple of good and seasonal fruits, taken perhaps as a mid-morning and afternoon snack.

5. Try to **find sweetness in other things in life**, such as love and affection.

6. Decide to **take time to learn at least one relaxation technique** that helps reduce stress and therefore the search for sugar. For example, mindfulness meditation and yoga are useful.

7. **Do not rely only on willpower:** it is too easy to think that you are strong enough to win all the battles, but it is better to recognize your weaknesses and try to organize planned rewards. After a week without sugar, for example, indulge in an ice cream. It is important to set deadlines but also to take one step at a time to try to

solve a problem. By doing so, the body will begin to reward you with sensations of greater energy, mental clarity and will perceive this reward giving life to a change that will be truly lasting over time because it is based on a feeling of greater well-being.

As with any change, exceeding a time threshold of about two months will help make the gesture automatic. The fatigue that an action requires in the beginning decreases over time with exposure, as the body and mind get used to the new condition and it becomes evident to the person that he can live well in the new context. Once automaticity is acquired, on a psychological level, not adopting the new behavior costs more effort than adopting it. For example, in those who have overcome the obstacle, the idea of putting sugar in coffee creates more disturbance than drinking it bitter. It is not miracle, innate personal tastes, luck, or genetics but simply habits that each of us can adopt with the right strategy.

In addition to the strategic decisions mentioned above, you always need a realization to change, called in technical terms "a corrective emotional experience". It is a time when, usually all of a sudden, a person realizes that the effort of staying as it is outweighs the effort required to change. Sometimes it is a real experience, others simply a shift of perspective that allows us to see the problem from another angle.

Think for a moment: is what you sacrifice today really much compared to the health you will have tomorrow? Do you prefer to remain at the mercy of the currents, weak, addicted to food or other vices that make up for what you lack in life or roll up your sleeves and become a leader from a victim?

It is not just about losing weight but really changing thanks to a path made up of small correct decisions taken every day.

Changing means preventing the serious illnesses of tomorrow and above all regaining our true health starting today.

Learn to protect your health through nutrition by protecting yourself from the damage of excess sugar.

CHAPTER 5:

Breakfast and Snacks

1. Cheesy Low-Carb Omelet

Preparation Time: 10 minutes
Cooking Time: 30 minutes
Servings: 2
Ingredients:

- 2 whole eggs
- 1 tbsp. water
- 1 tbsp. butter
- 3 thin slices of salami
- 5 fresh basil leaves
- 5 thin slices, fresh ripe tomatoes
- 2 oz. fresh mozzarella cheese
- Salt and pepper as needed

Directions:
1. Take a small bowl and whisk in eggs and water.
2. Take a nonstick Sauté pan and place it over medium heat, add butter and let it melt.
3. Pour egg mixture and cook for 30 seconds.
4. Spread salami slices on half of the egg mix and top with cheese, tomatoes, basil slices.
5. Season with salt and pepper according to your taste.
6. Cook for 2 minutes and fold the egg with the empty half.
7. Cover and cook on LOW for 1 minute.
8. Serve and enjoy!

Nutrition:
- **Calories:** 451
- **Carbs:** 3 g
- **Protein:** 33 g
- **Fat:** 36 g

2. Apple & Cinnamon Pancake

Preparation Time: 10 minutes
Cooking Time: 30 minutes
Servings: 2
Ingredients:

- ¼ tsp. ground cinnamon
- 1 ¾ cups better baking mix
- 1 tbsp. oil
- 1 cup water
- 2 egg whites
- ½ cup sugar-free applesauce
- Cooking spray
- 1 cup plain yogurt
- Sugar substitute

Directions:
1. Blend the cinnamon and the baking mix in a bowl.
2. Create a hole in the middle and add the oil, water, egg, and applesauce.
3. Mix well.
4. Spray your pan with oil.
5. Place it on medium heat.

6. Pour ¼ cup of the batter.
7. Flip the pancake and cook until golden.
8. Serve with yogurt and sugar substitute.

Nutrition:
- **Calories:** 231
- **Total carbs:** 37 g
- **Protein:** 8 g
- **Total fat:** 6 g
- **Saturated fat:** 1 g
- **Cholesterol:** 54 mg
- **Sodium:** 545 mg
- **Dietary fiber:** 4 g
- **Potassium:** 750 mg

3. Cream Cheese Pancakes

Preparation Time: 5 minutes
Cooking Time: 10 minutes
Servings: 2
Ingredients:

- ½ tsp. cinnamon
- 2 oz. cream cheese
- 1 tsp. maple sugar
- 2 eggs, large

Directions:
1. Place eggs, cream cheese, maple sugar, and cinnamon in a high-speed blender and blend until combined well. Set it aside for 2 minutes.
2. Heat a large-sized skillet over medium heat.
3. When the skillet becomes hot, spoon ¼ of the batter to it and spread it to a circle.
4. Cook for 2 to 3 minutes on each side until cooked. Flip it. Cook the other side for 1 minute.
5. Repeat with the remaining batter and serve.

Tip: Serve it along with sugar-free syrup or berries.

Nutrition:
- **Calories:** 344
- **Carbs:** 3 g
- **Proteins:** 17 g
- **Fat:** 29 g
- **Sodium:** 10 mg

4. Bulgur Porridge

Preparation Time: 10 minutes
Cooking Time: 30 minutes
Servings: 2
Ingredients:

- ⅔ cup unsweetened soy milk
- ⅓ cup bulgur, rinsed
- Pinch of salt
- 1 ripe banana, peeled and mashed
- 2 kiwis, peeled and sliced

Directions:
1. In a pan, add the soy milk, bulgur, and salt over medium-high heat and bring to a boil.
2. Adjust the heat to low and simmer for about 10 minutes.
3. Remove the pan of bulgur from heat and immediately, stir in the mashed banana.
4. Serve warm with the topping of kiwi slices.

Nutrition:
- **Calories:** 223
- **Total carbs:** 47.5 g
- **Protein:** 7.1 g
- **Total fat:** 2.3 g
- **Saturated fat:** 0.3 g
- **Cholesterol:** 0 mg
- **Sodium:** 126 mg
- **Fiber:** 8.6 g

5. Rhubarb Muffins

Preparation Time: 10 minutes
Cooking Time: 25 minutes
Servings: 2
Ingredients:

- ½ cup almond meal
- 2 tbsp. crystallized ginger
- ¼ cup coconut sugar
- 1 tbsp. linseed meal
- ½ cup buckwheat flour
- ¼ cup brown rice flour
- 2 tbsp. powdered arrowroot
- 2 tsp. gluten-free baking powder
- ½ tsp. freshly grated ginger
- ½ tsp. ground cinnamon
- 1 cup rhubarb, sliced
- 1 apple, cored, peeled, and chopped
- ⅓ cup almond milk, unsweetened
- ¼ cup olive oil
- 1 free-range egg
- 1 tsp. vanilla extract

Directions:

1. In a bowl, mix the almond meal with the crystallized ginger, sugar, linseed meal, buckwheat flour, rice flour, arrowroot powder, grated ginger, baking powder, and cinnamon; stir.
2. In another bowl, mix the rhubarb with the apple, almond milk, oil, egg, and vanilla and stir well.
3. Combine the 2 mixtures, stir well, and divide into a lined muffin tray. Place in the oven at 350° F and bake for 25 minutes. Serve the muffins for breakfast.
4. Enjoy!

Nutrition:

- Calories: 200
- Carbs: 13 g
- Protein: 8 g
- Fat: 4 g
- Fiber: 6 g

6. Turkey-Broccoli Brunch Casserole

Preparation Time: 10 minutes
Cooking Time: 30 minutes
Servings: 2
Ingredients:

- 2-½ cups turkey breast, cubed and cooked
- 16 oz. broccoli, chopped and drained
- 1-½ cups of milk, fat-free
- 1 cup cheddar cheese, low-fat, shredded
- 10 oz. cream of chicken soup (low sodium and low fat)

What you will need from the store cupboard:

- 8 oz. egg substitute
- ¼ tsp. poultry seasoning
- ¼ cup of sour cream, low fat
- ½ tsp. pepper
- ⅛ tsp. salt
- 2 cups of seasoned stuffing cubes
- Cooking spray

Directions:

1. Bring together the egg substitute, soup, milk, pepper, sour cream, salt, and poultry seasoning in a big bowl.

2. Now stir in the broccoli, turkey, ¾ cup of cheese, and stuffing cubes.
3. Transfer to a baking dish. Apply cooking spray.
4. Bake for 10 minutes. Sprinkle the remaining cheese.
5. Bake for another 5 minutes.
6. Keep it aside for 5 minutes. Serve.

Nutrition:
- Calories: 303
- Carbs: 26 g
- Protein: 33 g
- Total fat: 7 g
- Fiber: 3 g
- Cholesterol: 72 mg

7. Guacamole Turkey Burgers

Preparation Time: 10 minutes
Cooking Time: 30 minutes
Servings: 2
Ingredients:
- 12 oz. turkey, ground
- 1-½ avocados
- 2 tsp. of juice from a lime
- ½ tsp. cumin
- 1 red chili, chopped

What you will need from the store cupboard:
- ½ tsp. garlic powder
- ½ tsp. onion powder
- 3 tsp. olive oil
- ½ tsp. salt

Directions:
1. Mix the turkey with the cumin, chili, salt, garlic powder, and onion powder in a medium-sized bowl.
2. Create 3 patties.
3. Pour 3 tsp. of olive oil into a skillet and heat over medium heat.
4. Now cook your patties. Make sure that both sides are brown.
5. Make the guacamole in the meantime.
6. Mash together the garlic powder, juice from the lime, and avocados in a bowl.
7. Add salt for seasoning.
8. Serve the burgers with guacamole on the patties.

Nutrition:
- Calories: 316
- Carbs: 9 g
- Protein: 24 g
- Total fat: 21 g
- Fiber: 8 g
- Cholesterol: 80 mg

8. Ham and Goat Cheese Omelet

Preparation Time: 10 minutes
Cooking Time: 30 minutes
Servings: 2
Ingredients:
- 1 slice of ham, chopped
- 4 egg whites
- 2 tsp. water
- 2 tbsp. onion, chopped
- 1 tbsp. parsley, minced

What you will need from the store cupboard:
- 2 tbsp. green pepper, chopped
- ⅛ tsp. pepper
- 2 tbsp. goat cheese, crumbled
- Cooking spray

Directions:
1. Whisk together the water, pepper, and egg whites in a bowl till everything blends well.
2. Stir in the green pepper, ham, and onion.
3. Now heat your skillet over medium heat after applying the cooking spray.
4. Pour in the egg white mix towards the edge.
5. As it sets, push the cooked parts to the center. Allow the uncooked portions to flow underneath.
6. Sprinkle the goat cheese to one side when there is no liquid egg.
7. Now fold your omelet in half.
8. Sprinkle the parsley.

Nutrition:
- **Calories:** 143
- **Carbs:** 5 g
- **Protein:** 21 g
- **Total fat:** 4 g
- **Fiber:** 1 g
- **Cholesterol:** 27 mg

9. Breakfast Smoothie

Preparation Time: 15 minutes
Cooking Time: 0 minutes
Servings: 2
Ingredients:
- 1 cup frozen blueberries
- ½ cup pineapple chunks
- ½ cup english cucumber
- ½ apple
- ½ cup water

Directions:
1. Put the pineapple, blueberries, cucumber, apple, and water in a blender and blend until thick and smooth.
2. Pour into 2 glasses and serve.

Nutrition:
- **Calories:** 87
- **Carbs:** 22 g
- **Protein:** 0.7 g
- **Phosphorus:** 28 mg
- **Potassium:** 192 mg
- **Sodium:** 3 mg

10. Bagels

Preparation Time: 15 minutes
Cooking Time: 15 minutes
Servings: 2
Ingredients:
- 1 tbsp. baking powder
- 1 ½ cup almond flour, blanched
- 2 eggs, large & beaten
- 2 ½ cup mozzarella cheese, shredded
- 2 oz. cream cheese, cubed

Directions:
1. Preheat the oven to 400° F.
2. Combine almond flour and baking powder in a mixing bowl. Set aside.
3. Mix the mozzarella cheese and cream cheese in a large microwave-safe bowl and heat it for 2 minutes on high power. Stir halfway through and at the end.
4. Add the flour mixture and eggs to the cheese mixture and make a dough out of it by kneading it quickly.
5. As the dough will be sticky, keep kneading it until it becomes smooth. **Tip:** If the dough seems too

difficult to mix or is still sticky, you can microwave it again for another 15 to 20 seconds to make it soften.
6. Divide the dough into six portions and roll it into a long log.
7. Press the ends together of the long log to get the bagel shape. Arrange them on a parchment paper-lined baking sheet.
8. Finally, bake them for 12 to 14 minutes or until the bagels are firm and golden in color.

Tip: You can top it with sesame seeds if desired.

Nutrition:
- **Calories:** 360
- **Carbs:** 5 g
- **Proteins:** 21 g
- **Fat:** 28 g
- **Sodium:** 54 mg

11. Buckwheat and Grapefruit Porridge

Preparation Time: 5 minutes
Cooking Time: 20 minutes
Servings: 2
Ingredients:
- ½ cup buckwheat
- ¼ grapefruit, chopped
- 1 tbsp. honey
- 1 ½ cups almond milk
- 2 cups water

Directions:
1. Boil water on the stove. Add the buckwheat and place the lid on the pan.
2. Simmer for 7 to 10 minutes, in low heat. Check to ensure water does not dry out.
3. Remove and set aside for 5 minutes, do this when most of the water is absorbed.
4. Drain excess water from the pan and stir in almond milk, heating through for 5 minutes.
5. Add the honey and grapefruit.
6. Serve.

Nutrition:
- **Calories:** 231
- **Carb:** 43 g
- **Fat:** 4 g
- **Phosphorus:** 165 mg
- **Potassium:** 370 mg
- **Sodium:** 135 mg

12. Egg and Veggie Muffins

Preparation Time: 15 minutes
Cooking Time: 20 minutes
Servings: 2
Ingredients:
- Cooking spray
- 4 eggs
- 2 tbsp. unsweetened rice milk
- ½ sweet onion, chopped
- ½ red bell pepper, chopped
- ½ cup parsley
- Pinch red pepper flakes
- Pinch ground black pepper

Directions:
1. Preheat the oven to 350° F.
2. Spray 4 muffin pans with cooking spray. Set aside.
3. Whisk together the milk, eggs, onion, red pepper, parsley, red pepper flakes, and black pepper until mixed.

4. Pour the egg mixture into prepared muffin pans.
5. Bake until the muffins are puffed and golden, about 18 to 20 minutes. Serve

Nutrition:
- **Calories:** 84
- **Carb:** 3 g
- **Fat:** 5 g
- **Protein:** 7 g
- **Phosphorus:** 110 mg
- **Potassium:** 117 mg
- **Sodium:** 75 mg

13. Quinoa Congee With Cauliflower

Preparation Time: 5 minutes
Cooking Time: 20 minutes
Servings: 2
Ingredients:
- 6 cups water
- ¼ cup quinoa
- 4 large leeks, minced (reserve green stems for garnish)
- 1 small cauliflower head, minced
- 1 can mackerel in water, low-sodium, flaked (include liquid)
- 1 tbsp. fresh ginger, grated
- 1 tbsp. low-sodium teriyaki sauce, add more water only if needed
- ¼ lb. frozen scallops, thawed
- ½ lb. frozen shrimps, thawed
- Pinch of sea salt
- Pinch of white pepper
- 1 lime, sliced into wedges

Directions:
1. Except for lime, scallops, and shrimps, pour the remaining ingredients into a slow cooker set at low heat. Stir. Put the lid on. Cook for 6 hours. Stir in scallops and shrimps; cook for another 15 minutes. Turn off heat. **Taste:** adjust seasoning if needed.
2. Ladle congee into individual bowls. Garnish with leeks. Serve with a wedge of lime on the side. Squeeze lime juice into congee just before eating.

Nutrition:
- **Protein:** 10.11 g
- **Potassium:** 364 mg
- **Sodium:** Na 180 mg

14. Winter Fruit Salad

Preparation Time: 10 minutes
Cooking Time: 0 minutes
Servings: 2
Ingredients:
- 4 persimmons, cubed
- 4 pears, cubed
- 1 cup grapes, halved
- 1 cup apples, peeled, cored, and cubed
- ¾ cup pecans, halved
- 1 tbsp. olive oil
- 1 tbsp. peanut oil
- 1 tbsp. pomegranate flavored vinegar
- 2 tbsp. agave nectar

Directions:
1. In a salad bowl, mix the persimmons with the pears, grapes, apples, and pecans.

In another bowl, mix the olive oil with the peanut oil, vinegar, and agave nectar. Whisk well then pour over the salad, toss and serve for breakfast.
2. Enjoy!

Nutrition:
- **Calories:** 125 **Carbs:** 14 g
- **Protein:** 8 g **Fat:** 3 g
- **Fiber:** 6 g

Buckwheat Granola

Preparation Time: 10 minutes
Cooking Time: 45 minutes
Servings: 2
Ingredients:
- 2 cups oats
- 1 cup buckwheat
- 1 cup sunflower seeds
- 1 cup pumpkin seeds
- 1 ½ cups dates, pitted and chopped
- 1 cup apple puree
- 6 tbsp. coconut oil
- 5 tbsp. cocoa powder
- 1 tsp. freshly grated ginger

Directions:
1. In a large bowl, mix the oats with the buckwheat, sunflower seeds, pumpkin seeds, dates, apple puree, oil, cocoa powder, and ginger then stir really well. Spread on a lined baking sheet, press well, and place in the oven at 360° F for 45 minutes. Leave the granola to cool down, slice, and serve for breakfast.
2. Enjoy!

Nutrition:
- **Calories:** 161 **Carbs:** 11 g

- **Protein:** 7 g
- **Fat:** 3 g
- **Fiber:** 5 g

15. Mushroom Frittata

Preparation Time: 10 minutes
Cooking Time: 30 minutes
Servings: 2
Ingredients:
- ¼ cup coconut milk, unsweetened
- 6 eggs
- 1 yellow onion, chopped
- 4 oz. white mushrooms, sliced
- 2 tbsp. olive oil
- 2 cups baby spinach
- A pinch of salt and black pepper

Directions:
1. Heat up a pan with the oil over medium-high heat, add the onion, stir and cook for 2 to 3 minutes. Add the mushrooms, salt, and pepper, stir and cook for 2 minutes more. In a bowl, mix the eggs with coconut milk, salt and pepper, stir well and pour over the mushrooms. Add the spinach, mix a bit, place in the oven, and bake at 360° F for 25 minutes. Slice the frittata and serve it for breakfast.
2. Enjoy!

Nutrition:
- **Calories:** 200 **Carbs:** 14 g
- **Protein:** 6 g
- **Fat:** 3 g
- **Fiber:** 6 g

16. Breakfast Crepes

Preparation Time: 10 minutes
Cooking Time: 10 minutes
Servings: 2
Ingredients:

- 2 eggs -1 tsp. vanilla extract
- ½ cup almond milk, unsweetened
- ½ cup water
- 2 tbsp. agave nectar
- 1 cup coconut flour
- 3 tbsp. coconut oil, melted

Directions:

1. In a bowl, whisk the eggs with vanilla extract, almond milk, water, and agave nectar. Add the flour and 2 tbsp. of oil gradually and stir until you obtain a smooth batter. Heat up a pan with the rest of the oil over medium heat, add some of the batter, spread into the pan, and cook the crepe until it's golden on both sides then transfer to a plate. Repeat with the rest of the batter and serve the crepes for breakfast.
2. Enjoy!

Nutrition:

- **Calories:** 121 **Carbs:** 14 g
- **Protein:** 6 g **Fat:** 3 g
- **Fiber:** 6 g

17. Cherry Berry Bulgur Bowl

Preparation Time: 15 minutes.
Cooking Time: 15 minutes.
Servings: 2
Ingredients:

- 1 cup medium-grind bulgur
- 2 cups water
- Pinch salt
- 1 cup halved and pitted cherries or 1 cup canned cherries, drained
- ½ cup raspberries
- ½ cup blackberries
- 1 tbsp. cherry jam
- 2 cups plain whole-milk yogurt

Directions:

1. Mix the bulgur, water, and salt in a medium saucepan. Do this in medium heat. Bring to a boil.
2. Reduce the heat to low and simmer, partially covered, for 12 to 15 minutes or until the bulgur is almost tender. Cover, and let stand for 5 minutes to finish cooking do this after removing the pan from the heat.
3. While the bulgur is cooking, combine the raspberries and blackberries in a medium bowl. Stir the cherry jam into the fruit.
4. When the bulgur is tender, divide among four bowls. Top each bowl with ½ cup of yogurt and an equal amount of the berry mixture and serve.

Nutrition:

- **Calories:** 242
- **Carbs:** 44 g
- **Protein:** 9 g
- **Total fat:** 6 g
- **Saturated fat:** 3 g
- **Sodium:** 85 mg
- **Phosphorus:** 237 mg
- **Potassium:** 438 mg
- **Fiber:** 7 g

18. Citrus Blueberry Muffins

Preparation Time: 5 minutes
Cooking Time: 30 minutes
Servings: 2
Ingredients:

- 2 cups blueberries
- 2 tsp. phosphorus-free baking powder
- 1 tsp. lime zest
- 2 cups plain flour
- ½ cup light sour cream
- 1 tsp. lemon zest
- 1 cup unsweetened rice milk
- 2 eggs -1 cup coconut sugar
- ½ cup melted coconut oil

Directions:

1. Warm the oven to 400° F. Take a cupcake tin and place paper liners in each cup. Place the coconut sugar and coconut oil into a medium bowl. Using a hand mixer, beat until fluffy.
2. Add in sour cream, rice milk, and eggs. Scrape and continue to mix until well blended. Add baking powder, lime zest, lemon zest, and flour to a small bowl. Stir together to combine. Mix the flour mixture into the eggs until it just comes together. Add in the blueberries and stir again. Spoon into prepared muffin papers. Don't overfill. Place into the preheated oven and bake for 25 minutes.
3. Check to make sure a toothpick comes out clean when stuck to the muffins. Serve and enjoy!

Nutrition:

- **Calories:** 252 **Protein:** 4 g
- **Sodium:** 26 mg
- **Potassium:** 107 mg
- **Phosphorus:** 79 mg

19. Pineapple Bread

Preparation Time: 5 minutes
Cooking Time: 20 minutes
Servings: 2
Ingredients:

- ⅓ cup Swerve
- ⅓ cup butter, unsalted
- 2 eggs - 2 cups flour
- 3 tsp. baking powder
- 1 cup pineapple, undrained
- 6 cherries, chopped

Directions:

- Whisk the Swerve with the butter in a mixer until fluffy.
- Stir in the eggs, then beat again. Add the baking powder and flour, then mix well until smooth.
- Fold in the cherries and pineapple.
- Spread this cherry-pineapple batter in a 9x5 inch baking pan.
- Bake the pineapple batter for 1 hour at 350° F.
- Slice the bread and serve.

Nutrition:

- **Calories:** 197 **Carbs:** 18.3 g
- **Protein:** 4 g **Total fat:** 7.2 g
- **Saturated fat:** 1.3 g
- **Cholesterol:** 33 mg
- **Sodium:** 85 mg
- **Dietary fiber:** 1.1 g
- **Calcium:** 79 mg
- **Phosphorous:** 316 mg
- **Potassium:** 227 mg

20. Zucchini Bread

Preparation Time: 25 minutes
Cooking Time: 40 minutes
Servings: 2
Ingredients:

- ¾ cup shredded zucchini
- ½ cup almond flour
- ¼ tsp. salt
- ¼ cup cocoa powder, unsweetened
- ½ cup chocolate chips, unsweetened, divided
- 6 tbsp. maple syrup
- ½ tsp. baking soda
- 2 tbsp. olive oil
- ½ tsp. vanilla extract, unsweetened
- 2 tbsp. butter, unsalted, melted
- 1 egg, pastured

Directions:

1. Switch on the air fryer, insert the fryer basket, grease it with olive oil, then shut with its lid, set the fryer at 310° F, and preheat for 10 minutes.
2. Meanwhile, place flour in a bowl, add salt, cocoa powder, and baking soda, and stir until mixed.
3. Crack the eggs in another bowl, whisk in sweetener, egg, oil, butter, and vanilla until smooth, and then slowly whisk in flour mixture until incorporated.
4. Add zucchini along with ⅓ cup chocolate chips and then fold until just mixed.
5. Take a mini loaf pan that fits into the air fryer, grease it with olive oil, then pour in the prepared batter and sprinkle the remaining chocolate chips on top.
6. Open the fryer, place the loaf pan in it, close with its lid, and cook for 30 minutes at 310° F until inserted toothpick into the bread slides out clean.
7. When the air fryer beeps, open its lid, remove the loaf pan, then place it on a wire rack and let the bread cool in it for 20 minutes.
8. Take out the bread, let it cool completely, then cut it into slices and serve.

Nutrition:

- **Calories:** 356
- **Carbs:** 49 g
- **Fat:** 17 g
- **Protein:** 5.1 g
- **Fiber:** 2.5 g

21. Keto Scrambled Eggs

Preparation Time: 10 minutes
Cooking Time: 30 minutes
Servings: 2
Ingredients:

- 4 eggs, large
- 2 tbsp. scallions, sliced thinly
- 3 tbsp. butter
- ½ tsp. salt
- ⅓ cup heavy cream
- 2 tbsp. cilantro, chopped
- 1 serrano chili pepper
- Dash of pepper
- 1 tomato, small & chopped

Directions:

1. Melt the butter by heating a large non-stick pan over medium-high heat.

2. Once the pan is hot, stir in the chili and tomato to it and cook for 2 minutes.
3. Mix eggs, pepper, cilantro, cream, salt, and chili in a medium bowl with a whisker until combined well.
4. Pour the egg mixture into the pan and allow it to cook.
5. With a spatula, fold the edges toward the center. **Tip:** Allow the egg to set around the edges.
6. Continue cooking for a few more minutes or until soft.
7. Sprinkle with scallions.
8. Serve it hot.

Tip: You can add more low-carb veggies if preferred.

Nutrition:
- **Calories:** 455
- **Carbs:** 4 g
- **Proteins:** 14 g
- **Fat:** 43 g
- **Sodium:** 641 g

22. Strawberry & Spinach Smoothie

Preparation Time: 10 minutes
Cooking Time: 30 minutes
Servings: 2
Ingredients:
- 1 ½ cups fresh strawberries, hulled and sliced
- 2 cups fresh baby spinach
- ½ cup fat-free plain Greek yogurt
- 1 cup unsweetened almond milk
- ¼ cup ice cubes

Directions:
1. In a high-speed blender, add all the ingredients and pulse until smooth.
2. Pour into serving glasses and serve immediately.

Nutrition:
- **Calories:** 96
- **Total carbs:** 12.3 g
- **Protein:** 8.1 g
- **Total fat:** 2.3 g
- **Saturated fat:** 0.2 g
- **Cholesterol:** 1 mg
- **Fiber:** 3.9 g
- **Sodium:** 144 mg
- **Potassium:** 428 mg

23. Tomato and Zucchini Sauté

Preparation Time: 10 minutes
Cooking Time: 30 minutes
Servings: 2
Ingredients:
- 1 tbsp. vegetable oil
- 2 tomatoes (chopped)
- 1 green bell pepper (chopped)
- Black pepper, freshly ground, as per taste
- 1 onion (sliced)
- 2 lb. zucchini, peeled and cut into 1-inch-thick slices
- Salt, as per taste
- ¼ cup uncooked white rice

Directions:
1. Begin by getting a nonstick pan and putting it over low heat. Stream in the oil and allow it to heat through.
2. Put in the onion and sauté for about 3 minutes.
3. Then pour in the zucchini, tomato, and green pepper. Mix well and spice with black pepper and salt.
4. Reduce the heat and cover the pan with a lid. Allow the

veggies to cook on low for 5 minutes.
5. While you're done, put in the water and rice. Place the lid back on and cook on low for 20 minutes.

Nutrition:
- Calories: 94
- Carbs: 16.1 g
- Fat: 2.8 g
- Protein: 3.2 g

24. Banana Matcha Breakfast Smoothie

Preparation Time: 10 minutes
Cooking Time: 0 minutes
Servings: 2
Ingredients:
- 1 cup fat-free milk
- 1 medium banana, sliced
- ¼ cup frozen chopped pineapple
- ½ cup ice cubes
- 1 tbsp. matcha powder
- ¼ tsp. ground cinnamon
- Liquid stevia extract, to taste

Directions:
1. Combine the ingredients in a blender.
2. Pulse the mixture several times to chop the ingredients.
3. Blend for 30 to 60 seconds until smooth and well combined.
4. Sweeten to taste with liquid stevia extract, if desired.
5. Pour into a glass and serve immediately.

Nutrition:
- Calories: 230
- Total carbs: 44.9 g
- Net carbs: 38 g
- Protein: 12.6 g
- Total fat: 0.4 g
- Saturated fat: 0.1 g
- Fiber: 6.9 g
- Sodium: 135 mg

25. Tofu and Vegetable Scramble

Preparation Time: 10 minutes
Cooking Time: 30 minutes
Servings: 2
Ingredients:
- 16 oz. firm tofu (drained)
- ½ tsp. sea salt
- 1 tsp. garlic powder
- Fresh coriander, for garnishing
- ½ medium red onion
- 1 tsp. cumin powder
- Lemon juice, for topping
- 1 medium green bell pepper
- 1 tomato
- ¼ tsp. chili powder
- ¼ tsp. chili flakes
- ¼ tsp. turmeric powder

Directions:
1. Begin by preparing the ingredients. For this, you are to extract the seeds of the tomato and green bell pepper. Shred the onion, bell pepper, and tomato into small cubes.
2. Get a small mixing bowl and position the fairly hard tofu inside it. Make use of your hands to break the fairly hard tofu. Arrange aside.
3. Get a nonstick pan and add in the onion, tomato, and bell pepper. Mix and cook for about 3 minutes.

4. Put the somewhat hard crumbled tofu into the pan and combine well.
5. Get a small bowl and put in the water, turmeric, garlic powder, cumin powder, and chili powder. Combine well and stream it over the tofu and vegetable mixture.
6. Allow the tofu and vegetable crumble to cook with seasoning for 5 minutes. Continuously stir so that the pan is not holding the ingredients.
7. Drizzle the tofu scramble with chili flakes and salt. Combine well.
8. Transfer the prepared scramble to a serving bowl and give it a proper spray of lemon juice.
9. Finalize by garnishing with pure and neat coriander. Serve while hot!

Nutrition:
- **Calories:** 238
- **Carbs:** 16.6 g
- **Fat:** 11 g

26. Basil and Tomato Baked Eggs

Preparation Time: 10 minutes
Cooking Time: 30 minutes
Servings: 2
Ingredients:
- 1 garlic clove, minced
- 1 cup canned tomatoes
- ¼ cup fresh basil leaves, roughly chopped
- ½ tsp. chili powder
- 1 tbsp. olive oil
- 4 whole eggs
- Salt and pepper to taste

Directions:
1. Preheat your oven to 375° F.
2. Take a small baking dish and grease with olive oil.
3. Add garlic, basil, tomatoes chili, olive oil into a dish and stir.
4. Crack down eggs into a dish, keeping space between the two.
5. Sprinkle the whole dish with salt and pepper.
6. Place in oven and cook for 12 minutes until eggs are set and tomatoes are bubbling.
7. Serve with basil on top.
8. Enjoy!

Nutrition:
- **Calories:** 235
- **Carbs:** 7 g
- **Protein:** 14 g
- **Fat:** 16 g

27. Berry Breakfast Bark

Preparation Time: 10 minutes
Freeze Time: 2 hours
Cooking Time: 0 minutes
Servings: 6
Ingredients:
- 3 to 4 strawberries, sliced
- 1 ½ cup plain Greek yogurt
- ½ cup blueberries

What you'll need from the store cupboard:
- ½ cup low-fat granola
- 3 tbsp. sugar-free maple syrup

Directions:
1. Line a baking sheet with parchment paper.
2. In a medium bowl, mix yogurt and syrup until

combined. Pour into prepared pan and spread in a thin even layer.
3. Top with remaining ingredients. Cover with foil and freeze for 2 hours or overnight.

To serve:
1. Slice into squares and serve immediately. If bark thaws too much it will lose its shape. Store any remaining bark in an airtight container in the freezer.

Nutrition:
- **Calories:** 69
- **Total carbs:** 18 g
- **Net carbs:** 16 g
- **Protein:** 7 g
- **Fat:** 6 g
- **Fiber:** 2 g

28. Chia and Coconut Pudding

Preparation Time: 10 minutes
Cooking Time: 30 minutes
Servings: 2
Ingredients:
- 7 oz. light coconut milk
- 3 to 4 drops liquid stevia
- 1 kiwi
- ¼ cup chia seeds
- 1 clementine
- Shredded coconut (unsweetened)

Directions:
1. Begin by getting a mixing bowl and putting in the light coconut milk. Set in the liquid stevia to sweeten the milk. Combine well.
2. Put the chia seeds into the milk and whisk until well-combined. Arrange aside.
3. Scrape the clementine and carefully extract the skin from the wedges. Leave aside.
4. Also, scrape the kiwi and dice it into small pieces.
5. Get a glass vessel and gather the pudding. For this, position the fruits at the bottom of the jar; then put a dollop of chia pudding. Then spray the fruits and then put another layer of chia pudding.
6. Finalize by garnishing with the rest of the fruits and chopped coconut.

Nutrition:
- **Calories:** 201
- **Carbs:** 22.8 g
- **Protein:** 5.4 g
- **Fat:** 10 g

29. Apple Filled Swedish Pancake

Preparation Time: 25 minutes
Cooking Time: 20 minutes
Servings: 2
Ingredients:
- 2 apples, cored and sliced thin
- ¾ cup egg substitute
- ½ cup fat-free milk
- ½ cup sugar-free caramel sauce
- 1 tbsp. reduced-calorie margarine

What you'll need from the store cupboard:
- ½ cup flour
- 1-½ tbsp. coconut sugar

- 2 tsp. water
- ¼ tsp. cinnamon
- ⅛ tsp. cloves
- ⅛ tsp. salt
- Nonstick cooking spray

Directions:
1. Heat oven to 400° F. Place margarine in cast iron, or ovenproof, skillet and place in oven until margarine is melted.
2. In a medium bowl, whisk together flour, milk, egg substitute, cinnamon, cloves, and salt until smooth.
3. Pour batter in hot skillet and bake 20 to 25 minutes until puffed and golden brown.
4. Spray a medium saucepan with cooking spray. Heat over medium heat.
5. Add apples, coconut sugar, and water. Cook, stirring occasionally until apples are tender and golden brown, about 4 to 6 minutes.
6. Pour the caramel sauce into a microwave-proof measuring glass and heat 30 to 45 seconds, or until warmed through.
7. To serve, spoon apples into pancakes and drizzle with caramel. Cut into wedges.

Nutrition:
- **Calories:** 193
- **Total carb:** 25 g
- **Net carbs:** 23 g
- **Protein:** 6 g
- **Fat:** 2 g
- **Fiber:** 2 g

30. Apple Topped French Toast

Preparation Time: 10 minutes.
Cooking Time: 10 minutes.
Servings: 2
Ingredients:
- 1 apple, peel and slice thin
- 1 egg
- ¼ cup skim milk
- 2 tbsp. margarine, divided

What you'll need from the store cupboard:
- 4 slices healthy loaf bread
- 1 tbsp. stevia
- 1 tsp. vanilla
- ¼ tsp. cinnamon

Directions:
1. Melt 1 tbsp. of margarine in a large skillet over med-high heat. Add apples, stevia, and cinnamon and cook, stirring frequently, until apples are tender.
2. In a shallow dish, whisk together egg, milk, and vanilla.
3. Melt the remaining margarine in a separate skillet over med-high heat. Dip each slice of bread in the egg mixture and cook until golden brown on both sides.
4. Place two slices of French toast on plates, and top with apples. Serve immediately.

Nutrition:
- **Calories:** 394
- **Total carbs:** 27 g
- **Net carbs:** 22 g
- **Protein:** 10 g **Fat:** 23 g
- **Fiber:** 5 g

31. Bacon & Egg Muffins

Preparation Time: 10 minutes
Cooking Time: 15 minutes
Servings: 2
Ingredients:

- 1 ¼ cups frozen hash browns, thawed
- 1 cup egg substitute
- 2 turkey sausage patties, diced
- 2 tbsp. onion, diced fine
- 2 tbsp. turkey bacon, cooked and chopped
- 2 tbsp. Monterey Jack cheese, grated
- 1 tbsp. fat-free sour cream

What you'll need from the store cupboard:

- 1 clove garlic, diced fine
- 1 tsp. vegetable oil
- ¼ tsp. salt
- ⅛ tsp. black pepper

Directions:

1. Heat oven to 400° F. Spray a 6-cup muffin pan with cooking spray.
2. Divide the hash browns evenly among the muffin cups, pressing firmly on the bottoms and up the sides.
3. In a large skillet, over medium heat, heat oil until hot. Add onion, and cook stirring frequently until tender.
4. Add garlic and sausage and cook for 1 minute.
5. Remove the skillet from heat and stir in sour cream.
6. In a medium bowl, beat egg substitute with salt and pepper. Pour the egg mixture evenly over the potatoes. Top with sausage mixture, bacon, and cheese. Bake 15 to 18 minutes, or until eggs are set. Serve immediately.

Nutrition:

- **Calories:** 165
- **Total carbs:** 13 g
- **Net carbs:** 12 g
- **Protein:** 11 g
- **Fat:** 7 g **Fiber:** 1 g

32. Cauliflower Breakfast Hash

Preparation Time: 10 minutes
Cooking Time: 30 minutes
Servings: 2
Ingredients:

- 4 cups cauliflower, grated
- 1 cup mushrooms, diced
- ¾ cup onion, diced
- 3 slices bacon
- ¼ cup sharp cheddar cheese, grated

Directions:

1. In a medium skillet, over med-high heat, fry bacon, set aside.
2. Add vegetables to the skillet and cook, stirring occasionally, until golden brown.
3. Cut bacon into pieces and return to skillet.
4. Top with cheese and allow it to melt. Serve immediately.

Nutrition:

- **Calories:** 155
- **Total carbs:** 16 g
- **Net carbs:** 10 g
- **Protein:** 10 g
- **Fat:** 7 g **Fiber:** 6 g

33. Vegetable Frittata

Preparation Time: 10 minutes
Cooking Time: 20 minutes
Servings: 2
Ingredients:

- 8 eggs, large 2 tbsp. olive oil
- $2/3$ cup cheddar cheese
- 1 ½ cup mushrooms, sliced
- ¼ tsp. salt
- 1 cup bell peppers, sliced into strips
- ¼ tsp. black pepper
- 1 cup zucchini, sliced into quartered
- ¼ cup heavy cream

Directions:

1. Preheat the oven to 350° F.
2. Spoon oil to a heated cast-iron skillet over medium heat.
3. Stir in the vegetables and cook them for 4 to 6 minutes or until softened.
4. In the meantime, whisk eggs, salt, heavy cream, and pepper in a medium-sized bowl until combined well.
5. Add the egg mixture over the vegetables and add the cheese over it. Mix gently.
6. Transfer the cast-iron skillet to the oven and bake for 18 to 20 minutes or until the top is puffy while being just set in the middle.
7. Allow it to cool for 10 minutes before serving.

Tip: You can add your choice of low-carb veggies to it.

Nutrition:

- **Calories:** 188 **Carbs:** 1 g
- **Proteins:** 11 g **Fat:** 15 g
- **Sodium:** 223 g

34. Vegetable Omelet

Preparation Time: 15 minutes
Cooking Time: 10 minutes
Servings: 2
Ingredients:

- 4 egg whites
- 1 egg
- 2 tbsp. chopped fresh parsley
- 2 tbsp. water
- Olive oil spray
- ½ cup chopped and boiled red bell pepper
- ¼ cup chopped scallion, both green and white parts
- Ground black pepper

Directions:

1. Whisk together the egg, egg whites, parsley, and water until well blended. Set aside.
2. Spray a skillet with olive oil spray and place over medium heat.
3. Sauté the peppers and scallion for 3 minutes or until softened.
4. Over the vegetables, you can now pour the egg and cook, swirling the skillet, for 2 minutes or until the edges start to set. Cook until set.
5. Season with black pepper and serve.

Nutrition:

- **Calories:** 77
- **Carb:** 2 g
- **Protein:** 12 g
- **Fat:** 3 g
- **Phosphorus:** 67 mg
- **Potassium:** 194 mg
- **Sodium:** 229 mg

35. Mexican Style Burritos

Preparation Time: 5 minutes
Cooking Time: 15 minutes
Servings: 2
Ingredients:

- 1 tbsp. olive oil
- 2 corn tortillas
- ¼ cup red onion, chopped
- ¼ cup red bell peppers, chopped
- ½ red chili, deseeded and chopped
- 2 eggs
- Juice of 1 lime
- 1 tbsp. cilantro, chopped

Directions:
1. Turn the broiler to medium heat and place the tortillas underneath for 1 to 2 minutes on each side or until lightly toasted.
2. Remove and keep the broiler on.
3. Sauté onion, chili, and bell peppers for 5 to 6 minutes or until soft.
4. Place the eggs on top of the onions and peppers and place the skillet under the broiler for 5 to 6 minutes or until the eggs are cooked.
5. Serve half the eggs and vegetables on top of each tortilla and sprinkle with cilantro and lime juice to serve.

Nutrition:

- **Calories:** 202 **Carb:** 19 g
- **Protein:** 9 g **Fat:** 13 g
- **Phosphorus:** 184 mg
- **Potassium:** 233 mg
- **Sodium:** 77 mg

36. Fast Microwave Egg Scramble

Preparation Time: 5 minutes
Cooking Time: 1 to 2 minutes
Servings: 2
Ingredients:

- 1 large egg
- 2 large egg whites
- 2 tbsp. milk
- Kosher pepper, ground

Directions:
1. Spray a coffee cup with a bit of cooking spray.
2. Whisk all the ingredients together and place them into the coffee cup.
3. Place the cup with the eggs into the microwave and set to cook for approx. 45 seconds. Take out and stir.
4. Cook it for another 30 seconds after returning it to the microwave.
5. Serve.

Nutrition:

- **Calories:** 128.6
- **Carbs:** 2.47 g
- **Protein:** 12.96 g
- **Fat:** 5.96 g
- **Sodium:** 286.36 mg
- **Potassium:** 185.28 mg
- **Phosphorus:** 122.22 mg
- **Dietary Fiber:** 0 g

37. Bacon & Eggs

Preparation Time: 5 minutes
Cooking Time: 20 minutes
Servings: 2
Ingredients:

- 4 eggs, large
- 2 ½ oz. bacon, sliced

- Sprigs of parsley, fresh & chopped

Directions:
1. Heat a medium-sized pan over high heat, and once it becomes hot, fry the bacon in it until it becomes crispy. Set it aside on a plate and leave the fat in the pan.
2. Crack the eggs into the bacon grease.
3. Cook the eggs according to your preference.
4. Add salt and pepper as needed.
5. Serve it hot and top it with parsley.

Tip: If preferred, you can even top it with sliced cherry tomatoes.

Nutrition:
- **Calories:** 272
- **Carb:** 1 g
- **Proteins:** 15 g
- **Fat:** 22 g
- **Sodium:** 280 g

38. Summer Veggie Omelet

Preparation Time: 5 minutes
Cooking Time: 5 minutes
Servings: 2
Ingredients:
- 4 large egg whites
- ¼ cup of sweet corn, frozen
- ⅓ cup of zucchini, grated
- 2 green onions, sliced
- 1 tbsp. cream cheese
- Kosher pepper

Directions:
1. Grease a medium pan with some cooking spray and add the onions, corn, and grated zucchini.
2. Sauté for a couple of minutes until softened.
3. Beat the eggs together with the water, cream cheese, and pepper in a bowl.
4. Add the eggs into the veggie mixture in the pan, and let cook while moving the edges from inside to outside with a spatula, to allow raw egg to cook through the edges.
5. Turn the omelet with the aid of a dish (placed over the pan and flipped upside down and then back to the pan).
6. Let sit for another 1 to 2 minutes.
7. Fold in half and serve.

Nutrition:
- **Calories:** 90
- **Carbs:** 15.97 g
- **Protein:** 8.07 g
- **Fat:** 2.44 g
- **Sodium:** 227 mg
- **Potassium:** 244.24 mg
- **Phosphorus:** 45.32 mg
- **Dietary fiber:** 0.88 g

39. Sweet Pancakes

Preparation Time: 10 minutes
Cooking Time: 5 minutes
Servings: 2
Ingredients:
- 1 cup all-purpose flour
- 1 tbsp. maple sugar
- 2 tsp. baking powder
- 2 egg whites
- 1 cup almond milk
- 2 tbsp. olive oil
- 1 tbsp. maple extract

Directions:
1. Combine the flour, maple sugar, and baking powder in a bowl.
2. Make a well in the center and place it to one side.
3. Mix the egg whites, milk, oil, and maple extract, do this in another bowl.
4. Add the egg mixture to the well and gently mix until a batter is formed.
5. Heat skillet over medium heat.
6. Cook 2 minutes on each side or until the pancake is golden only add $1/5$ of the batter to the pan.
7. Repeat with the remaining batter and serve.

Nutrition:
- **Calories:** 178
- **Protein:** 6 g
- **Fat:** 6 g
- **Potassium:** 126 mg
- **Sodium:** 297 mg

40. Summer Breakfast Parfait

Preparation Time: 10 minutes
Cooking Time: 30 minutes
Servings: 2
Ingredients:
- 1 5-oz. container vanilla Greek yogurt
- 1 peach, sliced thin
- ¼ cup blueberries

What you'll need from the store cupboard:
- ⅓ cup granola

Directions:
1. Layer half the yogurt on the bottom of a glass or Mason jar. Top with half the granola, half the peach, and half the berries. Repeat. Eat immediately.

Nutrition:
- **Calories:** 78
- **Total carbs:** 20 g
- **Net carbs:** 17 g
- **Protein:** 6 g
- **Fat:** 6 g
- **Fiber:** 3 g

41. Cauliflower Potato Mash

Preparation Time: 10 minutes
Cooking Time: 30 minutes
Servings: 2
Ingredients:
- 2 cups potatoes, peeled and cubed
- 2 tbsp. butter
- ¼ cup milk
- 10 oz. cauliflower florets
- ¾ tsp. salt

Directions:
1. Add water to the saucepan and bring to boil.
2. Reduce heat and simmer for 10 minutes.
3. Drain vegetables well. Transfer vegetables, butter, milk, and salt to a blender and blend until smooth.

Nutrition:
- **Calories:** 128
- **Carbs:** 16.3 g
- **Protein:** 3.2 g **Fat:** 6.2 g
- **Cholesterol:** 17 mg

42. Garlic Bread

Preparation Time: 10 minutes
Cooking Time: 30 minutes
Servings: 2
Ingredients:

- 2 stale French rolls
- 4 tbsp. crushed or crumpled garlic
- 1 cup of mayonnaise
- Powdered grated parmesan
- 1 tbsp. olive oil

Directions:

1. Preheat the air fryer. Set the time of 5 minutes and the temperature to 200° C.
2. Mix mayonnaise with garlic and set aside.
3. Cut the baguettes into slices, but without separating them completely.
4. Fill the cavities of equals. Brush with olive oil and sprinkle with grated cheese.
5. Place in the basket of the air fryer. Set the timer to 10 minutes, adjust the temperature to 180° C, and press the power button.

Nutrition:

- **Calories:** 340 **Carbs:** 32 g
- **Protein:** 15 g
- **Fat:** 15 g
- **Cholesterol:** 0 mg

43. Fried Egg

Preparation Time: 10 minutes
Cooking Time: 30 minutes
Servings: 2
Ingredients:

- 1 egg, pastured
- 1/8 tsp. salt
- 1/8 tsp. cracked black pepper
- Olive oil

Directions:

1. Take the fryer pan, grease it with olive oil and then crack the egg in it.
2. Switch on the air fryer, insert the fryer pan, then shut with its lid, and set the fryer at 370° F.
3. Set the frying time to 3 minutes, then when the air fryer beep, open its lid and check the egg if the egg needs more cooking, then air fryer it for another minute.
4. Transfer the egg to a serving plate, season with salt and black pepper, and serve.

Nutrition:

- **Calories:** 90
- **Carbs:** 0.6 g
- **Protein:** 6.3 g
- **Fat:** 7 g
- **Fiber:** 0 g

44. Quick Breakfast Yogurt Sundae

Preparation Time: 10 minutes
Cooking Time: 30 minutes
Servings: 2
Ingredients:

- ¾ cup plain Greek yogurt
- ¼ cup mixed berries (blueberries, strawberries, blackberries)
- 2 tbsp. cashew, walnut, or almond pieces
- 1 tbsp. ground flaxseed
- 2 fresh mint leaves, shredded

Directions:

1. Pour the yogurt into a tall parfait glass and scatter the

top with the berries, cashew pieces, and flaxseed.
2. Sprinkle the mint leaves on top for garnish and serve chilled.

Nutrition:
- Calories: 238
- Carbs: 15.8 g
- Protein: 20.9 g
- Fat: 11.2 g
- Fiber: 4.1 g
- Sodium: 63 mg

45. Coconut Breakfast Porridge

Preparation Time: 10 minutes
Cooking Time: 30 minutes
Servings: 2
Ingredients:
- 4 cup vanilla almond milk, unsweetened
- Blueberries, to taste
- Honey, to taste

What you'll need from the store cupboard:
- 1 cup unsweetened coconut, grated
- 8 tsp. coconut flour

Directions:
1. Add coconut to a saucepan and cook over med-high heat until it is lightly toasted. Be careful not to let it burn.
2. Add milk and bring to a boil. While stirring, slowly add flour, cook, and stir until mixture starts to thicken about 5 minutes.
3. Remove from heat, mixture will thicken more as it cools. Ladle into bowls, add blueberries or drizzle with a little honey if desired.

Nutrition:
- Calories: 231
- Total carbs: 21 g
- Net carbs: 8 g
- Protein: 6 g
- Fat: 14 g
- Fiber: 13 g

46. Whole-Grain Pancakes

Preparation Time: 10 minutes
Cooking Time: 30 minutes
Servings: 2
Ingredients:
- 2 cups whole-wheat pastry flour
- 4 tsp. baking powder
- 2 tsp. ground cinnamon
- ½ tsp. salt
- 2 cups skim milk, plus more as needed
- 2 large eggs
- 1 tbsp. honey
- Nonstick cooking spray
- Maple syrup, for serving
- Fresh fruit, for serving

Directions:
1. In a large bowl, stir together the flour, baking powder, cinnamon, and salt.
2. Add the milk, eggs, and honey, and stir well to combine. If needed, add more milk, 1 tbsp. at a time, until there are no dry spots and you have a pourable batter.
3. Heat a large skillet over medium-high heat, and spray it with cooking spray.
4. Using a ¼-cup measuring cup, scoop 2 or 3 pancakes into the skillet at a time.

Cook for a couple of minutes, until bubbles form on the surface of the pancakes, flip, and cook for 1 to 2 minutes more, until golden brown and cooked through. Repeat with the remaining batter.
5. Serve topped with maple syrup or fresh fruit.

Nutrition:
- **Calories:** 392
- **Carbs:** 71 g
- **Protein:** 15 g
- **Total fat:** 4 g
- **Saturated fat:** 1 g
- **Fiber:** 9 g
- **Cholesterol:** 95 mg
- **Sodium:** 396 mg

47. Granola With Fruits

Preparation Time: 10 minutes
Cooking Time: 30 minutes
Servings: 2
Ingredients:
- 3 cups quick-cooking oats
- 1 cup almonds, sliced
- ½ cup wheat germ
- 3 tbsp. butter
- 1 tsp. ground cinnamon
- 1 cup honey
- 3 cups whole-grain cereal flakes
- ½ cup raisins
- ½ cup dried cranberries
- ½ cup dates, pitted and chopped

Directions:
1. Preheat your oven to 325° F.
2. Place the almonds on a baking sheet.
3. Bake for 15 minutes.
4. Mix the wheat germ, butter, cinnamon, and honey in a bowl.
5. Add the toasted almonds and oats.
6. Mix well.
7. Spread on the baking sheet.
8. Bake for 20 minutes.
9. Mix with the rest of the ingredients.
10. Let cool and serve.

Nutrition:
- **Calories:** 210
- **Total carbs:** 36 g
- **Protein:** 5 g
- **Total fat:** 7 g
- **Saturated fat:** 2 g
- **Cholesterol:** 5 mg
- **Sodium:** 58 mg
- **Dietary fiber:** 4 g
- **Potassium:** 250 mg

48. Egg Muffins

Preparation Time: 10 minutes
Cooking Time: 30 minutes
Servings: 2
Ingredients:
- 1 tbsp. green pesto
- 3 oz. / 75 g shredded cheese
- 5 oz. / 150 g cooked bacon
- 1 scallion, chopped
- 6 eggs
- Salt and pepper, to taste

Directions:
1. You should set your oven to 350°F / 175°C.
2. Place liners in a regular cupcake tin. This will help with easy removal and storage.
3. Beat the eggs with pepper, salt, and pesto. Mix in the cheese.

4. Pour the eggs into the cupcake tin and top with the bacon and scallion.
5. Cook for 15 to 20 minutes

Nutrition:
- **Calories:** 190
- **Carbs:** 4 g
- **Protein:** 7 g
- **Fat:** 15 g

49. Immunity Booster Smoothie

Preparation Time: 10 minutes
Cooking Time: 0 minutes
Servings: 2
Ingredients:
For the orange layer:
- 1 persimmon (quartered)
- 1 ripe mango (chopped)
- 1 lime (juiced)
- 1 tbsp. nut butter (of your choice)
- ½ tsp. turmeric powder
- 1 pinch of cayenne pepper
- 1 cup of coconut milk

For the pink layer:
- 1 small beet (cubed)
- 1 cup of berries (frozen)
- 1 pink grapefruit (quartered)
- ¼ cup of pomegranate juice
- ½ cup of water
- 6 leaves of mint
- 1 tsp. honey

Directions:
1. Add the ingredients for the orange layer in a blender. Blend for making a smooth liquid.
2. Pour the orange liquid evenly into serving glasses.
3. Add the pink layer ingredients to a blender. Blend for making a smooth liquid.
4. Pour the pink liquid slowly over the orange layer.
5. Pour in such a way so that both layers can be differentiated.
6. Serve immediately.

Nutrition:
- **Calories:** 301.9
- **Carbs:** 70.7 g
- **Protein:** 5.4 g
- **Fat:** 4.3 g
- **Fiber:** 8.9 g

CHAPTER 6:

First Courses

51. Healthier Egg Salad Sandwich

Preparation Time: 10 minutes
Cooking Time: 0 minutes
Servings: 2
Ingredients:

- 2 hard-cooked large eggs,
- 1 tbsp. fat-free sour cream
- 2 tsp. reduced-fat mayonnaise
- 2 slices reduced-fat whole-wheat bread
- ¼ tsp. Dijon-style mustard
- Pinch salt
- ¼ cup finely chopped celery
- Paprika for garnish

Directions:
1. Gently peel the eggs. Cut each egg in half. Carefully remove the yolks. Discard one yolk.
2. Mash the remaining egg yolk in a small bowl.
3. Add the sour cream, pickle relish, mayonnaise, mustard, and salt (if desired). Stir to mix well. Stir in the celery. Chop the egg whites and stir them into the yolk mixture.
4. Spread the mixture on each slice of bread. If desired, garnish with a light sprinkling of paprika.
5. Serve as open-faced sandwiches or place one on top of the other if you are packing up to take to work.

Nutrition:

- **Calories:** 100
- **Carbs:** 2.06 g
- **Protein:** 6.89 g
- **Fat:** 6.94 g

52. Sunday's Sausage Sandwich

Preparation Time: 15 minutes
Cooking Time: 17 to 20 minutes
Servings:
Ingredients:

- 1 lb. extra lean ground beef
- ½ lb. ground turkey breast
- 8 small Kaiser Rolls
- ¼ cup plain bread crumbs
- ½ cup skim milk
- 1/2 tsp. garlic powder
- 1 ½ tsp. dried oregano leaves
- 1 tsp. fennel seed, crushed
- 1 tsp. crushed red pepper flakes
- 1 large onion, halved, thinly sliced
- 1 large green bell pepper, seeded, thinly sliced
- 1 tbsp. water

Directions:
1. In a large bowl, combine ground beef, ground turkey, bread crumbs, milk, oregano, fennel, garlic powder, and crushed red pepper.
2. Mix well. Shape mixture into 8 patties, ½ inch thick.
3. Spray a large non-stick skillet with non-stick cooking spray. Heat over medium heat until hot.
4. Add onion, bell pepper and water then cover and cook for 5 minutes, stirring occasionally, or until vegetables are crisp-tender.
5. Remove veggies from skillet and cover to keep warm.
6. Wipe skillet clean and spray again with cooking spray. Heat over medium heat until hot.
7. Add patties and cook for about 12 minutes or until there is no pink in the center. Serve patties and veggies on Kaiser Rolls. Top with barbecue sauce if you want great while watching the game.

Nutrition:
- **Calories:** 727
- **Carbs:** 69.09 g
- **Protein:** 53.07 g
- **Fat:** 24.87 g

53. Mexican Style Tortillas With Pork

Preparation Time: 10 minutes
Cooking Time: 5 minutes
Servings: 4
Ingredients:
- 8 oz. lean boneless pork, cut into thin bite-size strips
- 4 8-inch whole-grain tortillas (to make fewer adjust the recipe)
- 1 tbs. olive oil
- 1 clove minced garlic
- ½ cup frozen whole kernel corn, thawed
- ½ cup chopped bottled roasted red sweet peppers
- ¼ cup sliced green onions
- 3 tbs. lime juice
- ½ tsp. ground cumin
- ⅛ tsp. cayenne pepper (optional)
- ½ cup canned refried black beans
- ½ cup shredded romaine lettuce
- ½ cup chopped tomatoes

Directions:
1. In a large skillet, heat oil over medium-high heat. Add pork and garlic and cook for 4 to 5 minutes or until pork is cooked through and juices run clear, stirring occasionally. Set aside.
2. Stir together the corn, roasted red peppers, green onions, 2 tbsp. of the lime juice, the cumin in a medium bowl. Add cayenne pepper (optional).
3. Mix the refried black beans and the remaining lime juice in a small bowl.
4. Spread 2 tbsp. of the black bean mixture in a 2-inch-wide strip down the center of each tortilla. Top with pork, corn mixture, lettuce, and tomatoes.

5. Fold the bottom edge of each tortilla over the filling to prevent spilling. Gently roll the tortillas around the filling.

Nutrition:
- **Calories:** 223
- **Carbs:** 23.24 g
- **Protein:** 19.35 g
- **Fat:** 6.37 g

54. Veggie Pasta Primavera

Preparation Time: 10 minutes
Cooking Time: 15 minutes
Servings: 4
Ingredients:
- 5 oz. multigrain pasta
- 1 tbsp. olive oil
- 1 tbsp. freshly minced garlic
- ½ cup minced spring onion
- ½ cup bell pepper
- ½ cup white kidney beans
- ½ tsp. lemon zest
- ½ tsp. lemon juice
- 1 cup fresh thyme leaves (½ tsp. dried thyme will also work)
- ½ cup white wine
- ½ cup concentrated vegetable broth (chicken broth will also do)
- 1 to 2 oz. parmesan (freshly grated is best)
- 1 tbsp. low salt butter
- Salt and pepper to taste

Directions:
1. Boil water for the multigrain pasta. Cover the pot! Use the instruction on the packet. Remember to follow the instructions for the letter. Multigrain pasta has a slightly different cooking time than the unhealthy kind.
2. While waiting, sauté some of the ingredients. Start by adding the cooking oil. Add the onions first. Wait several seconds, then add the garlic. A pinch of salt and pepper is needed at this point. Add the white kidney beans, next to the white wine, bell pepper, and thyme, broth, etc. Cover the pan.
3. By this time your water should be boiling. Add the pasta.
4. Go back to the veggies. Uncover the pan then stir fry for 3 to 5 minutes. You want your veggies to be half cooked. Turn off the heat, then add the butter on top.
5. Wait for the pasta to cook. Sample it to make sure it's just right. Strain then top with the vegetable. You want the pasta to be slightly undercooked when you drain off the water. The residual heat from the pasta and veggies should do the rest. Top it off with some freshly grated parmesan and some more thyme.
6. If you want, you can add a few slivers of bacon or pancetta to the mix! But that is only if it is your cheat day!

Nutrition:
- **Calories:** 396
- **Carbs:** 18.48 g
- **Protein:** 5.5 g
- **Fat:** 35.29 g

55. Meat Pasties

Preparation Time: 30 minutes
Cooking Time: 60 minutes
Servings: 12
Ingredients:
Dough:

- ½ cup trans-fat-free shortening
- ½ tsp. salt
- 2 cups all-purpose flour
- 7 tbsp. fat-free milk, or more

Filling:

- ¾ lb. 90%-lean ground beef
- 1 tbsp. chopped bell pepper
- 1 tbsp. chopped celery
- 1 tsp. dried basil
- 1 tsp. dried oregano
- 2 tbsp. barbecue sauce, lowest sodium available
- 2 tbsp. chopped onion

Directions:

1. Mix all ingredients for the dough and mix thoroughly. Put in as much milk as needed to make a soft dough.
2. Separate the dough into four parts. Roll each part out thin and cut into three 6-inch circles for a total of 12.
3. Mix all filling ingredients in a frying pan and cook until meat has browned.
4. Place 1 tbsp. of meat on each circle. Moisten edges of dough with water and fold in half to make a turnover. Seal edges well with a fork. Prick top to allow steam to escape. Place on unoil-coated cookie sheet.
5. Bake at 375° F for 40 minutes. Serve hot or cold.

Nutrition:

- **Calories:** 135
- **Total carb:** 18 g
- **Protein:** 8 g
- **Total fat:** 3 g
- **Cholesterol:** 15 mg
- **Sodium:** 140 mg
- **Potassium:** 145 g
- **Dietary fiber:** 1 g
- **Phosphorus:** 80 g

56. Stuffed Portobello Mushrooms

Preparation Time: 10 minutes
Cooking Time: 30 minutes
Servings: 4
Ingredients:

- 4 large portobello mushroom caps
- ¼ tsp. salt
- 1 cup part-skim ricotta cheese
- ½ cup finely shredded Parmesan cheese, divided
- ¼ tsp. freshly ground pepper, divided
- 1 cup finely chopped fresh spinach
- 2 tbs. finely chopped Kalamata olives
- ½ tsp. Italian seasoning
- ¾ cup prepared marinara sauce

Directions:

1. Preheat oven to 450° F. Coat a rimmed baking sheet with cooking spray.
2. Place mushroom caps, gill-side up, on the prepared pan.

Sprinkle with salt and ⅛ tsp. pepper. Roast the mushrooms until they are tender, usually about 20 to 25 minutes.
3. Place the ricotta spinach, ¼ cup Parmesan, olives, Italian seasoning, and the remaining ⅛ tsp. pepper in a medium bowl and mash them together until smooth.
4. Heat marinara sauce over low heat until hot.
5. Once the mushrooms are tender, carefully pour out any liquid accumulated in the caps and then return them to the pan gill-side up.
6. Spoon one tbs. marinara into each cap.
7. Mound a generous ⅓ cup ricotta filling into each cap and sprinkle with the remaining ¼ cup Parmesan. Bake until hot, about 10 minutes. Serve with the remaining marinara sauce.

Nutrition:
- **Calories:** 160
- **Carbs:** 8.94 g
- **Protein:** 11.63 g
- **Fat:** 8.94 g

57. Grilled Halibut With Veggies

Preparation Time: 10 minutes
Cooking Time: 30 minutes
Servings: 4
Ingredients:
- 1 lb. halibut (2 to 3 pieces)
- 1 tbsp. capers chopped
- 1 tbsp. spring onions
- Sea salt
- Fresh ground pepper
- 1 tsp. chopped almonds (optional)
- ½ cup slow-roasted halved and pitted cherry tomatoes (ordinary tomatoes will do)
- 3 pieces kalamata olives (pitted and chopped).
- 1 tbsp. vinaigrette or red wine vinegar
- 1 tbsp. olive oil (virgin and extra virgin will also do)

Directions:
1. Preheat the oven to 200° F (94° C).
2. First, you need to slow roast the cherry tomatoes. Wash, halve, and pit the same. Use ½ tbsp. of olive oil to pan-fry the olive halves. Remove after 5 minutes and transfer to a roasting dish. Sprinkle with a little bit of salt and pepper. Now place the tomatoes inside the oven and cook for 10 to 15 minutes or until the skin separates from the flesh, is wrinkly, and has small patches of charring. Let cool
3. Mix the tomatoes, olives, capers, vinaigrette in a bowl. Set aside.
4. Preheat a heavy cast-iron skillet. Add the olive oil and wait for it to smoke just a little bit. While waiting, lightly coat the halibut olive oil. Add salt and pepper. The oil keeps the salt and pepper on the halibut. And that dry rub keeps the halibut from sticking to the pan.
5. Cook the halibut. Depending on the thickness

of the halibut, it should cook for 5 to 6 minutes on each side. Don't overcook it; otherwise, the fish will turn tough and rubbery.
6. **Tip:** Look to the sides and the indentions on the curvature of the fillet. It should all turn a slightly opaque color.
7. Turn off the heat, wait 1 minute, and then plate. This way you don't peel off the outer layer of the halibut. Top with the tapenade and serve. If you are feeling festive, you can add a glass of your favorite white wine.

Nutrition:
- **Calories:** 252
- **Carbs:** 1.43 g
- **Protein:** 16.68 g
- **Fat:** 19.57 g

58. Burgoo

Preparation Time: 16 minutes
Cooking Time: 60 minutes
Servings: 16
Ingredients:

- 2 lb. pork butt, chopped into 1-inch pieces
- 2 lb. beef stew meat, chopped into 1-inch pieces
- 1 lb. boneless, skinless chicken thighs, chopped into 1-inch pieces
- 1 tsp. cayenne pepper
- 1 tsp. not old bay seasoning
- 3 cups chicken broth or store-bought low-sodium chicken broth
- 2 lb. potatoes, cut into 1-inch cubes
- 3 onions, chopped
- 2 green bell peppers, chopped
- 4 carrots, peeled and chopped
- 2 cups frozen corn
- 1 lb. okra, cut into 1-inch rounds
- 2 celery stalks, roughly chopped
- 1 cup frozen lima beans
- 2 large tomatoes, chopped
- 2 tbsp. tomato paste
- ¼ large cabbage, roughly chopped

Directions:
1. In an electric pressure cooker, combine the pork, beef, chicken, cayenne, and seasoning.
2. Cover with the broth, close and lock the lid, and set the pressure valve to sealing.
3. Select the Manual/Pressure Cook setting, and cook for 20 minutes.
4. Once cooking is complete, allow the pressure to release naturally. Carefully remove the lid.
5. Remove the meat, and shred with 2 forks.
6. To the pressure cooker, add the potatoes, onions, peppers, carrots, corn, okra, celery, lima beans, tomatoes, tomato paste, and cabbage. Close and lock the lid and set the pressure valve to sealing.
7. Select the Manual/Pressure Cook setting, and cook for 10 minutes.
8. Once cooking is complete, allow the pressure to release naturally. Carefully remove the lid.

9. Return the meat to the pressure cooker, change to the Sauté setting, and cook for 5 minutes, uncovered, or until the flavors meld.

Nutrition:
- **Calories:** 354
- **Protein:** 36 g
- **Fat:** 12 g

59. Mexican Beef Stew

Preparation Time: 15 minutes
Cooking Time: 90 minutes
Servings: 6
Ingredients:
- 1 cup onion, diced
- 1 ½ lb. beef round steak, sliced into ½-inch pieces
- 1 ¾ cups tomatoes, diced
- 1 cup carrots, diced
- ¼ cup sweet red pepper, diced
- 2 tbsp. cilantro, diced
- 1 jalapeno, seeded and diced
- 2 tbsp. flour
- 2 tbsp. water
- 1 ¾ cups low-sodium beef broth
- 1 garlic clove, diced
- ½ tsp. sea salt
- 1 ½ tbsp. chili powder
- 1 tbsp. vegetable oil

Directions:
1. Heat your oil in a pot over medium-high heat. Add the steak and cook until brown.
2. Add the broth, onion, carrots, red pepper, jalapeno, garlic, and seasonings, and bring to a boil. Reduce your heat to low and cover, then simmer for 45 minutes.
3. Stir stew occasionally.
4. Add your tomatoes and continue to cook for 15 minutes.
5. Stir the flour and water together in a bowl until smooth.
6. Add to your stew with the cilantro, then continue to cook for an additional 30 minutes; or until the stew has thickened.
7. Serve!

Nutrition:
- **Calories:** 312
- **Protein:** 39 g
- **Fat:** 13 g

60. Italian Veggie Soup

Preparation Time: 16 minutes
Cooking Time: 4 hours
Servings: 8
Ingredients:
- 4 cups cabbage, chopped
- 1 cup green beans, sliced into 1-inch pieces
- 2 cups fresh spinach, chopped
- 1 small onion, diced
- 2 green bell peppers, diced
- 2 celery stalks, diced
- 28 oz. can tomato, low-sodium, diced
- 6 cups low-sodium vegetable broth
- 1 tbsp. parsley
- 2 tbsp. tomato paste
- 1 ½ tsp. Italian seasoning
- 2 bay leaves
- 2 garlic cloves, fine diced
- 1 tbsp. basil
- Pepper to taste

Directions:
1. Add your vegetables to a crockpot.
2. Add the canned tomatoes, tomato paste, broth, bay leaves, Italian seasoning, and pepper and stir to combine.
3. Cover with a pot lid and cook on high for 5 hours. Add the basil, spinach, and parsley and cook for another additional 5 minutes.

Nutrition:
- Calories: 85
- Protein: 3 g
- Fats: 1 g

61. Korean Beef Soup

Preparation Time: 16 minutes
Cooking Time: 4 hours
Servings: 8
Ingredients:
- 1 gallon water
- 1 tbsp. oil
- 3 tbsp. soy sauce
- 1 tbsp. sesame seeds, toasted
- 2 garlic cloves, diced fine
- 1 tsp. sea salt
- 1 tsp. black ground pepper
- 1 lb. Beef, cubed
- 1 Korean white radish, peeled and diced
- 1 cup green onions, diced

Directions:
1. Set the crockpot to high and add the water.
2. In a mixing bowl, mix the soy sauce, green onions, sesame seeds, garlic, oil, sea salt, and pepper. Divide evenly between 2 Ziploc bags.
3. Place the meat in 1 bag and the radish in the other and allow to sit for 1 hour.
4. Turn the crockpot down to low and add the contents of the meat bag. Let cook for 1 hour, then add the contents of the radish bag. Cook for another 3 to 4 hours.

Nutrition:
- **Calories:** 120
- **Protein:** 19 g
- **Fats:** 4 g

62. Bell Pepper Stew

Preparation Time: 20 minutes
Cooking Time: 4 hours
Servings: 8
Ingredients:
- 3 cups onion, diced
- 3 cups green pepper, diced
- 1 lb. Hot Italian sausage, chopped
- 3 ½ cups tomatoes, diced
- 1 cup cauliflower, grated
- 1 lb. Lean ground sirloin
- 4 cups low-sodium beef broth
- 4 garlic cloves, fine diced
- 2 tbsp. olive oil
- 1 cup tomato sauce
- ½ tsp. oregano
- 1 tsp. basil

Directions:
1. Heat your oil in a large skillet over medium-high heat.
2. Add your onions and peppers to the pan and cook until tender.
3. Add your Italian chopped sausage to the pan and continue to cook for about

5 minutes or until the sausage is cooked.
4. Add remaining ingredients to crockpot, along with cooked sausage, onion, and peppers. Cook on high for 4 hours. Serve hot and enjoy!

Nutrition:
- **Calories:** 212
- **Protein:** 28 g
- **Fats:** 6 g

63. She-Crab Soup

Preparation Time: 16 minutes
Cooking Time: 25 minutes
Servings: 6
Ingredients:
- 2 cups seafood broth (here)
- 1 shallot, chopped
- 2 celery stalks, chopped
- 1 garlic clove, minced
- 1 tsp. not old bay seasoning
- 1 cup fat-free milk
- ½ cup half-and-half
- 1 tsp. hot sauce
- 1 tsp. Worcestershire sauce
- 1 1/8 lb. backfin lump crab meat
- 1 bunch chives, chopped
- Freshly ground black pepper
- Lemon wedges

Directions:
1. In a heavy-bottomed stockpot, bring the broth to a simmer.
2. Add the shallot, celery, garlic, and seasoning and cook for 3 to 5 minutes, or until softened.
3. Reduce the heat to low, and whisk in the milk, half-and-half, hot sauce, and Worcestershire sauce. Simmer for 10 minutes.
4. Add the crab and cook for 5 to 7 minutes, or until the flavors come together.
5. Serve with chives, pepper, and lemon wedges.

Nutrition:
- **Calories:** 116
- **Protein:** 16 g
- **Fat:** 4 g

64. Sweet Potato and Pumpkin Soup With Peanuts

Preparation Time: 10 minutes
Cooking Time: 45 minutes
Servings: 8
Ingredients:
- 3 cups vegetable broth (here) or store-bought low-sodium vegetable broth, divided
- 1 celery stalk, roughly chopped
- 1 cup roughly chopped tomato
- 1 red bell pepper, chopped
- 1 large sweet potato, peeled and cut into 2-inch cubes
- 1 small pumpkin, peeled and cut into 2-inch cubes
- 1 bay leaf
- 1 tsp. paprika
- 2 cups roasted unsalted peanuts
- Baby sage leaves (optional)

Directions:
1. In a large Dutch oven, bring 1 cup broth to a simmer over medium heat.
2. Add the celery, tomato, and bell pepper and cook for 5

to 7 minutes, or until softened.
3. Add the sweet potato, pumpkin, bay leaf, paprika, and the remaining 2 cups broth. Cover and cook for 30 minutes, or until the sweet potato and pumpkin are soft.
4. Add the peanuts and cook for 5 minutes, or until the peanuts become less crunchy. Discard the bay leaf.
5. Transfer to a heat-safe blender and pulse until the soup has a batter-like consistency.
6. Serve with grilled hearts of romaine with buttermilk dressing and protein of your choice. If using, garnish with baby sage leaves.

Nutrition:
- **Calories:** 266 **Protein:** 12 g
- **Fat:** 18 g

65. Spicy Chicken Stew

Preparation Time: 16 minutes
Cooking Time: 21 minutes
Servings: 8
Ingredients:
- 3 cups chicken broth or store-bought low-sodium chicken broth
- 6 boneless, skinless chicken breasts
- 1 tbsp. blackened rub
- 2 carrots, peeled and cut into 1-inch rounds
- 1 onion, roughly chopped
- 2 celery stalks, roughly chopped
- 1 medium sweet potato, cut into 1-inch chunks
- 2 cups fresh peas
- 2 cups roughly chopped green beans
- 2 garlic cloves, minced
- 1 cup chopped tomatoes
- 1 tbsp. tomato paste

Directions:
1. Select the Sauté setting on an electric pressure cooker and combine the broth, chicken, and rub. Cook for 5 minutes, or until the exterior of the chicken is lightly browned.
2. Add the carrots, onion, celery, sweet potato, peas, green beans, garlic, tomatoes, and tomato paste.
3. Close and lock the lid and set the pressure valve to sealing. Change to the Manual/Pressure Cook setting, and cook for 15 minutes at high pressure.
4. Once cooking is complete, quick-release the pressure. Carefully remove the lid, and serve.

Nutrition:
- **Calories:** 145
- **Protein:** 22 g
- **Fat:** 1 g

66. Tomato-Based Stew

Preparation Time: 16 minutes
Cooking Time: 61 minutes
Servings: 8
Ingredients:
- 5 cups chicken broth or store-bought low-sodium chicken broth, divided

- 1 medium onion, roughly chopped
- 2 garlic cloves, minced
- 4 boneless, skinless chicken thighs, roughly cut into chunks
- 3 sun-dried tomatoes, drained and roughly chopped
- 2 cups fresh lima beans
- 1 cup fresh corn kernels
- 1 zucchini, cut into 1-inch chunks
- 1 cup barbecue sauce
- 1 tbsp. Worcestershire sauce
- ½ tsp. not old bay seasoning

Directions:
1. Select the Sauté setting on an electric pressure cooker and combine 1 cup broth, onion, and garlic and cook for 1 to 2 minutes, or until the onion and garlic are translucent.
2. Add the chicken, sun-dried tomatoes, lima beans, corn, zucchini, and barbecue sauce, remaining 4 cups broth, the Worcestershire sauce, and seasoning.
3. Close and lock the lid and set the pressure valve to sealing.
4. Change to the Manual/Pressure Cook setting, and cook for 1 hour at high pressure.
5. Once cooking is complete, quick-release the pressure. Carefully remove the lid, and serve.

Nutrition:
- **Calories:** 262
- **Protein:** 22 g
- **Fat:** 4 g

67. Down South Corn Soup

Preparation Time: 10 minutes
Cooking Time: 35 minutes
Servings: 8
Ingredients:

- 1 tbsp. extra-virgin olive oil
- ½ Vidalia onion, minced
- 2 garlic cloves, minced
- 3 cups chopped cabbage
- 1 small cauliflower, broken into florets, or 1 (10 oz.) bag frozen cauliflower
- 1 (10 oz.) bag frozen corn
- 1 cup vegetable broth (here) or store-bought low-sodium vegetable broth
- 1 tsp. smoked paprika
- 1 tsp. ground cumin
- 1 tsp. dried dill
- ½ tsp. freshly ground black pepper
- 1 cup plain unsweetened cashew milk

Directions:
1. In a large stockpot, heat the oil over medium heat.
2. Add the onion and garlic, and sauté, stirring to prevent the garlic from scorching, for 3 to 5 minutes, or until translucent.
3. Add the cabbage and a splash of water, cover, and cook for 5 minutes, or until tender.
4. Add the cauliflower, corn, broth, paprika, cumin, dill, and pepper. Cover and cook for 20 minutes, or until tender.
5. Add the cashew milk and stir well. Cover and cook for

5 minutes, letting the flavors come together.
6. Serve with a heaping plate of greens and seafood of your choice.

Nutrition:
- **Calories:** 120
- **Protein:** 3 g
- **Fat:** 4 g

68. Carrot Soup

Preparation Time: 16 minutes
Cooking Time: 25 minutes
Servings: 6
Ingredients:

- 4 cups vegetable broth (here) or store-bought low-sodium vegetable broth, divided
- 2 celery stalks, halved
- 1 small yellow onion, roughly chopped
- ½ fennel bulb, cored and roughly chopped
- 1 (1-inch) piece fresh ginger, peeled and chopped
- 1 lb. carrots, peeled and halved
- 2 tsp. ground cumin
- 1 garlic clove, peeled
- 1 tbsp. almond butter

Directions:
1. Select the Sauté setting on an electric pressure cooker and combine ½ cup of broth, celery, onion, fennel, and ginger. Cook for 5 minutes, or until the vegetables are tender.
2. Add the carrots, cumin, garlic, remaining 3 ½ cups of broth, and almond butter.
3. Close and lock the lid, and set the pressure valve to sealing.
4. Change to the Manual/Pressure cook setting and cook for 15 minutes.
5. Once cooking is complete, quick-release the pressure. Carefully remove the lid, and let cool for 5 minutes.
6. Using a stand mixer or an immersion blender, carefully purée the soup. Serve with a heaping plate of greens.

Nutrition:
- **Calories:** 82
- **Protein:** 3 g
- **Fat:** 2 g

69. Bean Field Stew

Preparation Time: 20 minutes
Cooking Time: 41 minutes
Servings: 8
Ingredients:

- 6 cups vegetable broth (here) or store-bought low-sodium vegetable broth
- 1 cup dried lima beans
- 1 cup dried black beans
- 1 cup dried pinto beans
- 1 cup dried kidney beans
- 1 cup roughly chopped tomato
- 2 carrots, peeled and roughly chopped
- 1 zucchini, chopped
- ½ cup chopped white onion
- 1 celery stalk, roughly chopped
- 2 garlic cloves, minced
- 1 tsp. dried oregano
- 1 tsp. dried thyme

- ¼ tsp. freshly ground black pepper

Directions:
1. In an electric pressure cooker, combine the broth, lima beans, black beans, pinto beans, kidney beans, tomato, carrots, zucchini, onion, celery, garlic, oregano, thyme, and pepper.
2. Close and lock the lid and set the pressure valve to sealing.
3. Select the Manual/Pressure cook setting, and cook for 40 minutes.
4. Once cooking is complete, quick-release the pressure. Carefully remove the lid.
5. Serve with barbecue chicken.

Nutrition:
- **Calories:** 298
- **Protein:** 19 g
- **Fat:** 1 g

70. Pasta Salad

Preparation Time: 15 minutes
Cooking Time: 15 minutes
Servings: 4
Ingredients:
- 8 oz. whole-wheat pasta
- 2 tomatoes
- 1 (5-oz) pkg spring mix
- 9 slices bacon
- ⅓ cup mayonnaise (reduced-fat)
- 1 tbsp. Dijon mustard
- 3 tbsp. apple cider vinegar
- ¼ tsp. salt
- ½ tsp. pepper

Directions:
1. Cook pasta.
2. Chilled pasta, chopped tomatoes, and spring mix in a bowl.
3. Crumble-cooked bacon over pasta.
4. Combine mayonnaise, mustard, vinegar, salt, and pepper in a small bowl.
5. Pour dressing over pasta, stirring to coat.
6. Understanding diabetes is the first step in curing.

Nutrition:
- **Calories:** 200
- **Carbs:** 6 g
- **Protein:** 15 g
- **Fat:** 3 g

71. Chicken, Strawberry, and Avocado Salad

Preparation Time: 10 minutes
Cooking Time: 5 minutes
Servings: 4
Ingredients:
- 1,5 cups chicken (skin removed)
- ¼ cup almonds
- 2 (5-oz) pkg salad greens
- 1 (16-oz) pkg strawberries
- 1 avocado
- ¼ cup green onion
- ¼ cup lime juice
- 3 tbsp. extra virgin olive oil
- 2 tbsp. honey
- ¼ tsp. salt
- ¼ tsp. pepper

Directions:
1. Toast almonds until golden and fragrant.
2. Mix lime juice, oil, honey, salt, and pepper.

3. Mix greens, sliced strawberries, chicken, diced avocado, and sliced green onion, and sliced almonds; drizzle with dressing. Toss to coat.

Nutrition:
- **Calories:** 150
- **Carbs:** 5 g
- **Protein:** 15 g
- **Fat:** 10 g

72. Lemon-Thyme Eggs

Preparation Time: 10 minutes
Cooking Time: 5 minutes
Servings: 6
Ingredients:
- 7 large eggs
- ¼ cup mayonnaise (reduced-fat)
- 2 tsp. lemon juice
- 1 tsp. Dijon mustard
- 1 tsp. chopped fresh thyme
- ⅛ tsp. cayenne pepper

Directions:
1. Bring eggs to a boil.
2. Peel and cut each egg in half lengthwise.
3. Remove yolks to a bowl. Add mayonnaise, lemon juice, mustard, thyme, and cayenne to egg yolks; mash to blend. Fill egg white halves with yolk mixture.
4. Chill until ready to serve.

Nutrition:
- **Calories:** 40
- **Carbs:** 2 g
- **Protein:** 10 g
- **Fat:** 6 g

73. Spinach Salad with Bacon

Preparation Time: 15 minutes
Cooking Time: 0 minutes
Servings: 4
Ingredients:
- 8 slices center-cut bacon
- 3 tbsp. extra virgin olive oil
- 1 (5-oz) pkg. baby spinach
- 1 tbsp. apple cider vinegar
- 1 tsp. Dijon mustard
- ½ tsp. honey
- ¼ tsp. salt
- ½ tsp. pepper

Directions:
1. Mix vinegar, mustard, honey, salt, and pepper in a bowl.
2. Whisk in oil. Place spinach in a serving bowl; drizzle with dressing, and toss to coat.
3. Sprinkle with cooked and crumbled bacon.

Nutrition:
- **Calories:** 110
- **Carbs:** 1 g
- **Protein:** 6 g
- **Fat:** 2 g

74. Dijon Roasted Brussels Sprouts

Preparation Time: 10 minutes
Cooking Time: 30 minutes
Servings: 6
Ingredients:
- ¼ cup extra virgin olive oil
- 2 Tbsp Dijon mustard
- 2 Tbsp honey
- 1 Tbsp gluten free tamari
- 2 tsp dried tarragon

- 1 Tbsp Earth Balance soy free spread
- 2 lbs. Brussels sprouts, cored and quartered

Directions:
1. Whisk the first six ingredients together in medium size bowl.
2. Toss in Brussels sprouts to coat evenly.
3. Lay the sprouts in a baking sheet, rotating and stirring the sprouts after 15 minutes.
4. Put it back to the oven then roast again over 10 to 5 minutes.

Nutrition:
- Calories: 70
- Carbs: 14g
- Fat: 0g
- Protein: 5g

75. Quinoa Stuffing

Preparation Time: 10 minutes
Cooking Time: 15 minutes
Servings: 4
Ingredients:

- 2 Tbsp extra virgin olive oil
- ⅓ cup sliced leeks
- 2 cups cooked quinoa
- ½ tsp sea salt
- ¼ cup chopped cashews
- ¼ cup chopped unsulphured dried apricots
- ½ cup shredded kale
- 1 Tbsp maple syrup
- 1 Tbsp coconut aminos
- 1 tsp lemon zest
- 2 tsp dried thyme
- ½ tsp dried sage

Directions:
1. Warm-up olive oil in large skillet over medium heat.
2. Sauté leeks until softened and pour into a bowl.
3. Put the rest of the ingredients and season to taste with salt and pepper.
4. Serve warm or at room temperature.

Nutrition:
- Calories: 283
- Carbs: 49g
- Fat: 7g
- Protein: 6g

76. Italian Rice Bites

Preparation Time: 10 minutes
Cooking Time: 30 minutes
Servings: 10
Ingredients:

- 2 cups cooked brown rice
- Powdered egg replacer for 1 egg
- 3 Tbsp ground flax mixed with
- 1 Tbsp warm water
- 1 small onion, diced
- 4 cloves of garlic, minced
- ½ cup fresh basil, chiffonade
- ⅓ cup diced tomatoes
- ⅓ diced artichokes
- ½ cup vegan shredded mozzarella cheese
- 1 tsp ground fennel
- ½ tsp sea salt
- 2 Tbsp extra virgin olive oil
- ¼ cup nutritional yeast
- Pasta sauce, for dipping

Directions:
1. Warm-up oven to 425°F.
2. Mix the cooked rice with remaining ingredients, except pasta sauce in a large bowl; mix well to combine.

Scoop into greased muffin tins and press down with back of spoon. Bake within 25 minutes. Transfer from the oven; set aside to cool for 10 minutes. Serve with pasta sauce for dipping.

Nutrition:
- Calories: 120
- Carbs: 19g
- Fat: 4g
- Protein: 3g

77. Southwestern Sweet Bake

Preparation Time: 10 minutes
Cooking Time: 20 minutes
Servings: 4
Ingredients:

- 2 Tbsp extra virgin olive oil
- ¼ cup water
- 2 cups peeled sweet potato, sliced
- ½ cup sliced onion
- ½ red pepper, diced
- 1 jalapeno, diced finely
- ½ cup sliced shiitake mushrooms
- 2 cloves garlic, minced
- ½ cup unsweetened plain coconut milk yogurt
- ½ cup shredded vegan cheese
- ½ cup cashew cream (from extras section)
- 1 Tbsp ground cumin
- 1 tsp chili powder
- 1 tsp sea salt
- 1 avocado, diced
- ½ cup fresh cilantro leaves, chopped
- ½ cup salsa
- 10 organic corn tortilla chips, crushed

Directions:
1. Warm-up the oil and water in a medium sauté pan over medium high heat.
2. Add sweet potato, onions, red bell pepper and jalapeno and cook until sweet potatoes soften a bit, stirring occasionally for 5 to 7 minutes.
3. Stir in mushrooms and garlic and cook for 2 more minutes.
4. Stir in yogurt, cheese, cashew cream, cumin, chili powder and salt. Pour into casserole dish and bake at 400°F until bubbly, about 10 minutes.
5. Top with diced avocado, cilantro, salsa, and tortilla chips.

Nutrition:
- Calories: 290
- Carbs: 24g
- Fat: 22g
- Protein: 23g

78. Rice Pilaf

Preparation Time: 10 minutes
Cooking Time: 35 minutes
Servings: 5
Ingredients:

- 3 Tbsp Earth Balance soy free spread
- 1 shallot, thinly sliced
- ¼ cup finely chopped carrot
- 1 ½ tsp sea salt
- ½ tsp ground black pepper
- 1 ½ cups basmati brown rice
- ½ cup wild rice

- 1 ½ cups vegetable broth
- 1 ½ cups water
- 1 bay leaf
- 1 sprig fresh rosemary
- ½ cup dried cranberries
- 2 Tbsp maple syrup

Directions:
1. Melt the Earth Balance with the shallot and carrots in a medium saucepan over medium heat. Put salt and pepper then cook until the shallots and carrots are soft. Add the brown and wild rice and stir until coated with the Earth Balance. Adjust the heat to medium-high then allow the rice to toast for about 3 to 4 minutes, stirring occasionally.
2. Stir in the broth, water, bay leaf, and rosemary. Simmer over low heat setting, cover, and cook about 20 to 25 minutes. Transfer and let set for 5 minutes. Remove the rosemary and bay leaf. Fluff the rice with a fork, add cranberries and maple syrup and serve.

Nutrition:
- Calories: 105
- Carbs: 22g Fat: 1g
- Protein: 2g

79. Warm German Potato Salad

Preparation Time: 10 minutes
Cooking Time: 10 minutes
Servings: 6
Ingredients:
- 1 lb. baby red potatoes, cut into chunks
- ½ lb. green beans, cut into 2-inch pieces
- 2 Tbsp white balsamic vinegar
- ¼ cup vegan mayonnaise
- 2 Tbsp grainy mustard
- ¼ cup chopped fresh parsley
- 2 Tbsp chopped fresh dill
- 2 Tbsp chopped pimento peppers
- ½ tsp sea salt
- ¼ tsp black pepper
- 6 small scallions, chopped

Directions:
1. In a boiling salted water cook the potatoes within 8 minutes, or until tender. Add green beans during last minute of cooking. Strain potatoes and green beans then place in a large bowl.
2. Mix vinegar, mayonnaise, mustard, parsley, dill, pimento peppers, sea salt and black pepper in a small bowl. Stir until well combined. Pour over potatoes and beans, add scallions, and toss to coat.

Nutrition:
- Calories: 166
- Carbs: 18g
- Fat: 10g Protein: 2g

80. Roasted Cauliflower with Apple and Dill

Preparation Time: 10 minutes
Cooking Time: 40 minutes
Servings: 4
Ingredients:
- 1 cauliflower

- ½ large onion
- 1 large unpeeled apple
- 3 Tbsp extra virgin olive oil
- ¾ tsp sea salt
- 3 Tbsp dried cranberries
- ¼ cup plus 2 Tbsp coarsely chopped dill weed

Directions:
1. Warm-up oven to 425°F.
2. Put the cauliflower, onion, apple, olive oil, plus sea salt in a large deep baking dish then spread the fixing out into a single layer. Bake within 20 to 30 minutes, mixing occasionally. Stir in the cranberries and continue to bake within 10 more minutes, mixing from time to time. Serve with the dill, stir again before serving.

Nutrition:
- Calories: 105
- Carbs: 21g
- Fat: 3g
- Protein: 3g

81. Vegetarian Baked Beans

Preparation Time: 5 days
Cooking Time: 12 hours
Servings: 12
Ingredients:

- 3 cups dried navy beans
- 3 cups vegetable broth
- 1 - 6 oz. can tomato paste
- 1 Tbsp Worcestershire sauce
- ¼ cup brown sugar
- 2 Tbsp maple syrup
- 2 Tbsp molasses (not blackstrap)
- 2 Tbsp dried mustard
- 2 garlic cloves, minced
- ¼ cup sautéed chopped onion
- 2 tsp sea salt
- ¼ tsp black pepper

Directions:
1. Soak the beans 5 days before making beans, making certain to drain, rinse and refill the beans twice each day.
2. Drain beans and rinse off. Put beans into slow cooker. Add all the remaining ingredients and stir. Cover and cook within 12 hours on low. Serve.

Nutrition:
- Calories: 136
- Carbs: 30g
- Fat: 2g
- Protein: 4g

82. Jicama and Veggie Salad

Preparation Time: 15 minutes
Cooking Time: 0 minutes
Servings: 6
Ingredients:

Salad Ingredients:
- 1 lb. jicama, peeled and cubed
- 1 cup green beans, chopped
- 1 shallot, thinly sliced
- ¼ cup finely diced red onion
- ½ tsp sea salt
- 1 cup corn
- 1 large seedless cucumber, diced
- 1 roasted red bell pepper, diced
- 1 avocado, diced

- ½ cup sliced almonds
- 1 cup kidney beans, drained and rinsed
  Dressing:
- 6 oz. plain unsweetened coconut milk yogurt
- ¼ cup vegan mayonnaise
- 2 Tbsp coconut or apple cider vinegar
- 1 clove garlic, minced
- ¼ cup extra virgin olive oil
- Salt and freshly ground pepper, to taste
- 2-3 Tbsp fresh dill, chopped
- ¼ cup fresh parsley, chopped

Directions:
1. Mix all salad fixing in a large bowl.
2. Top with dressing (whisk all ingredients together). Toss to coat. This salad is best when chilled overnight.

Nutrition:
- Calories: 80
- Carbs: 6g
- Fat: 6g
- Protein: 2g

83. Broccoli Cheese Casserole

Preparation Time: 15 minutes
Cooking Time: 45 minutes
Servings: 6
Ingredients:

- 2 - 10 oz. packages frozen chopped broccoli
- 1 small onion, diced
- 4 Tbsp Earth Balance soy free spread
- 2 Tbsp sweet rice flour
- ½ cup water or coconut milk
- 1 cup cheese
- 3 beaten eggs
- ½ cup crushed gluten free crackers or breadcrumbs

Directions:
1. Warm-up the oven to 325°F.
2. Cook broccoli according to package instructions. Meanwhile, sauté onions in Earth Balance until soft. Whisk in sweet rice flour. Add water.
3. Cook over low heat setting, until thick and the batter comes to a boil. Stir in "cheese". Add beaten eggs.
4. Drain broccoli well and stir into sauce and eggs until blended. Bake with crumbs for 40 to 45 minutes.

Nutrition:
- Calories: 318
- Carbs: 10g
- Fat: 0g
- Protein: 0g

84. Italian Bean & Broccoli Sauté

Preparation Time: 15 minutes
Cooking Time: 15 minutes
Servings: 4
Ingredients:

- 2 Tbsp extra virgin olive oil
- 1 small red onion, sliced
- 3 cloves garlic, crushed
- 2 Tbsp tomato paste
- 2 cups broccoli
- 1 cup vegetable stock
- 2 cups kale, roughly chopped
- 2 cups spinach, roughly chopped

- ½ cup fresh cherry or grape tomatoes
- 1 – 15 oz. can cannellini beans
- 1 Tbsp fresh thyme
- 1 Tbsp fresh oregano
- ¼ cup fresh basil
- ½ teaspoon salt
- Pepper to taste

Directions:
1. Warm-up the olive oil in a sauté pan, and then add onions, garlic and tomato paste. Sauté until onions begin to soften.
2. Add broccoli and stock, cover pan, and steam until broccoli is tender and water is gone.
3. Add kale, spinach and tomatoes and sauté one minute.
4. Add beans and fresh herbs and continue to simmer until flavors meld together and beans are warm.
5. Add salt and pepper to taste.
6. Garnish with extra virgin olive oil and enjoy.

Nutrition:
- Calories: 57
- Carbs: 7g
- Fat: 2g
- Protein: 5g

85. Roasted Roots & Fruits with Creamy Balsamic Drizzle

Preparation Time: 15 minutes
Cooking Time: 40 minutes
Servings: 6
Ingredients:
- 1 red onion, sliced thinly
- 1 parsnip, peeled and diced
- 1 zucchini, sliced
- 1 rutabaga, peeled and diced
- 1 celery root, peeled and diced
- 6 Tbsp extra virgin olive oil, divided
- 1 cup grapes, halved
- 2 small pears, quartered
- ¼ cup walnut halves
- 1 avocado
- ¼ cup extra virgin olive oil
- ¼ cup balsamic vinegar
- 1 Tbsp Dijon mustard
- 2 tsp dried thyme
- 1 clove garlic
- 1 shallot, minced
- 1 tsp sea salt
- ½ tsp black pepper

Directions:
1. Warm-up the oven to 425°F.
2. Place the onion, parsnip, zucchini, rutabaga, and celery root on baking sheet. Grease with 3 tablespoons of olive oil then place in oven. Bake for 25 minutes, remove and add the grapes and pears. Bake for an additional 15 minutes. Remove from oven, sprinkle with walnuts and set aside.
3. In a blender, blend the avocado, 3 tablespoons of olive oil, balsamic vinegar, mustard, thyme, garlic, shallot, sea salt and pepper on high speed until creamy and thick. Drizzle over veggies.

Nutrition:
- Calories: 235
- Carbs: 54g Fat: 1g
- Protein: 3g

86. Cherry Tomatoes On The Side

Preparation Time: 5 minutes
Cooking Time: 5 minutes
Servings: 6
Ingredients:

- 1 tablespoon olive oil
- 2 pints cherry tomatoes
- 1/4 teaspoon sea salt
- 1/8 teaspoon freshly ground black pepper
- 2 teaspoons chopped fresh thyme leaves
- 1/4 cup freshly grated Parmesan cheese

Directions:

1. Heat the oil in skillet over medium-high heat. Add the tomatoes to the pan and season with salt and pepper. Sauté for 4–5 minutes, moving the tomatoes around the pan several times.
2. Toss the thyme on top and mix carefully with a spoon. Remove with a slotted spoon, sprinkle with Parmesan, and serve immediately.

Nutrition:

- Calories 9cal
- Carbs 1g Protein 0g

87. Ham And Asparagus Rolls With Cheese

Preparation Time: 5 minutes
Cooking Time: 25 minutes
Servings: 6
Ingredients:

- 1 bunch frozen asparagus
- 1/2-pound smoked ham, sliced thin
- 1/2-pound white American cheese, sliced thin

Directions:

1. Preheat oven to 350°F. Butter a 13" × 9" glass baking pan.
2. Place the frozen asparagus in boiling water within 1 minute and dry on paper towels. Put the slices of ham. Next is the slice of cheese and then an asparagus spear on each ham slice. Roll up and secure with toothpicks if necessary.
3. Place the rolls in the prepared pan. Pour the cheese sauce over the top. Bake within 25 minutes or until lightly browned on top and heated through. Serve hot.

Nutrition:

- Calories 80.5
- Total Fat 3.7 g
- Cholesterol 21.6 mg
- Sodium 472.0 mg
- Potassium 198.6 mg
- Total Carbohydrate 2.1 g
- Protein 9.7 g

88. Creamy Cheddar Sauce With Ham And Sherry

Preparation Time: 5 minutes
Cooking Time: 5 minutes
Servings: 21
Ingredients:

- 3 tablespoons unsalted butter
- 3 tablespoons corn flour

- 2 cups milk or heavy cream, warmed
- 2/3 cup grated sharp Cheddar cheese
- 1/4 cup minced smoked ham
- 2 teaspoons sherry
- 1/4 teaspoon salt
- 1/4 teaspoon ground black pepper

Directions:
1. Melt the butter then combine in the flour over medium-low heat mode. Sauté, stirring for 4–5 minutes. Put the warm milk or cream, whisking constantly until thickened to desired consistency.
2. Transfer then stir in the cheese, ham, sherry, and salt and pepper. Serve.

Nutrition:
- 83 Calories
- 4g Fat
- 10g Carbs
- 2g Protein

89. Crispy Potato Pancakes

Preparation Time: 5 minutes
Cooking Time: 5 minutes
Servings: 12
Ingredients:

- 6 potatoes, peeled and coarsely grated
- 2 mild onions, chopped fine
- 2 eggs, well beaten
- 1/2 cup potato flour
- 1 teaspoon salt
- 1/4 teaspoon ground black pepper
- Sour cream, applesauce, fruit preserves, salsa, or chutney to garnish

Directions:
1. Warm 1/2" olive oil in a skillet over medium heat and spoon in the potato cakes, pressing down to make patties.
2. Fry until golden brown, about 5 minutes per side. Drain, keep warm, and serve with garnish of choice.
3. Combine the grated potatoes, onions, eggs, potato flour, salt, and pepper in a mixing bowl.

Nutrition:
- 370 Calories
- 35g Carbs
- 24g Fat
- 4g Protein

90. Scalloped Potatoes With Leeks And Country Ham

Preparation Time: 35 minutes
Cooking Time: 90 minutes
Servings: 6
Ingredients:

- 1 1/2 cups grated Parmesan cheese
- 1 cup coarsely grated Fontina cheese
- 1/2 cup corn flour
- 1/4 teaspoon salt
- 1/4 teaspoon ground black pepper
- 6 Idaho or Yukon gold potatoes
- 4 leeks, thinly sliced
- 1-pound deli ham, diced
- 3 cups whole milk

- 4 tablespoons butter, divided

Directions:
1. Preheat oven to 350°F. Butter a 13" × 9" glass baking pan.
2. In a medium bowl, combine the cheeses, corn flour, salt, and pepper.
3. Put a layer of potatoes within the baking dish, then sprinkle 1/4 of the leeks and 1/4 of the ham on top. Sprinkle with 1/4 of the cheese mixture. Put the milk and dot with the butter.
4. Bake for approximately 90 minutes. Serve.

Nutrition:
- Calories 482.2
- Total Fat 28.3 g
- Total Carbohydrate 41.9 g
- Protein 15.9 g

91. Basic Cream Sauce

Preparation Time: 5 minutes
Cooking Time: 10 minutes
Servings: 2
Ingredients:
1. 3 tablespoons unsalted butter
2. 3 tablespoons corn flour
3. 2 cups whole milk
4. 1/4 teaspoon salt
5. 1/4 teaspoon ground black pepper
6. 1/8 teaspoon ground nutmeg, 1 teaspoon Dijon mustard, or 1 tablespoon snipped fresh chives (optional)

Directions:
1. Melt the butter then combine in the flour. Sauté, stirring for 4–5 minutes.
2. Put the warm milk or cream, whisking constantly until thickened to desired consistency.
3. Just before serving, add the salt and pepper. The optional fixing can be added at this time.

Nutrition:
- Calories 280.0
- Total Fat 4.0 g
- Cholesterol 20.0 mg
- Sodium 520.0 mg
- Potassium 340.0 mg
- Total Carbohydrate 51.0 g
- Protein 10.0 g

92. Parmesan-Crusted Asparagus

Preparation Time: 5 minutes
Cooking Time: 15 minutes
Servings: 8
Ingredients:
- 2 cups grated Parmesan cheese, divided
- 1 cup gluten-free Italian seasoned bread crumbs
- 2 tablespoons butter, melted
- 1/2 teaspoon salt
- 1/4 teaspoon ground black pepper
- 3 egg whites (from large eggs)
- 1 tablespoon coconut sugar
- 2 pounds thick asparagus spears, washed and trimmed

Directions:
1. Grease a baking sheet with olive oil.
2. Put 1 1/2 cups Parmesan, bread crumbs, butter, salt, and pepper in a 9" × 13" baking pan.
3. Whisk both egg whites and coconut sugar until soft peaks form. Put the asparagus and toss. Dig each spear in the bread crumb mixture and place on the prepared baking sheet.
4. Bake for 6–8 minutes or until just starting to brown. Sprinkle with the remaining Parmesan cheese and finish baking until the cheese is melted, about 5 minutes. Plate and serve immediately.

Nutrition:
- Calories 129.2
- Total Fat 5.8 g
- Total Carbohydrate 10.8 g
- Protein 10.1 g

93. Southern Cheese Grits

Preparation Time: 25 minutes
Cooking Time: 50 minutes
Servings: 10
Ingredients:
- 8 cups water
- 1/2 cup butter
- 2 cups quick-cooking grits
- 2 large eggs, lightly beaten
- 4 cups shredded sharp Cheddar cheese
- 1 teaspoon salt
- 1/2 teaspoon ground black pepper
- 1 tablespoon garlic powder
- 1/4 cup grated Parmesan cheese

Directions:
1. Preheat oven to 350°F. Grease a baking dish with butter.
2. Boil the water in an oven within medium-high heat. Whisk in the butter and grits. Decrease heat to low mode then simmer while whisking occasionally for 5–7 minutes.
3. Remove then stir 1 cup of grits into the eggs. Put the egg batter to the pot. Put the Cheddar cheese, salt, pepper, and garlic powder and stir.
4. Put the grits into the prepared pan then drizzle with the Parmesan cheese. Bake within 40 minutes or until the mixture is set and starts to turn golden brown. Serve and enjoy!

Nutrition:
- Calories: 282
- Carbs: 26g
- Fat: 14g
- Protein: 13g.

94. Italian Ricotta-Chestnut Fritters

Preparation Time: 60 minutes
Cooking Time: 5 minutes
Servings: 4
Ingredients:
- 2 large eggs
- 1 teaspoon baking soda
- 1 cup gluten-free ricotta cheese such as Organic Valley
- 1/2 cup chestnut flour
- 1/2 cup rice flour

Directions:
1. In a medium bowl, beat both eggs and sugar until stiff.
2. Slowly put the rest of the fixing. Let it sit for 1 hour.
3. Heat 2" of oil over medium-high heat in a deep-frying pan. Drop the batter by tablespoons into the oil. Do not overfill the pan. Fry within 2 minutes.

Nutrition:
- 408 Cal
- 15g Carbs
- 27g Fat
- 21g Protein

95. Home Fries

Preparation Time: 30 minutes
Cooking Time: 70 minutes
Servings: 6-8
Ingredients:

- 4 potatoes, washed and diced
- 2 teaspoons salt
- 2 tablespoons olive oil

Directions:
1. Preheat oven to 400°F. Grease a baking sheet with olive oil.
2. Meanwhile, put the diced potatoes in a 3-quart pot of water and boil within medium-high heat. Boil for exactly 7 minutes. Drain immediately in a colander and shake them around to roughen up the edges.
3. Place the boiled potatoes out onto the prepared baking sheet and drizzle with the olive oil. Sprinkle with Salt.
4. Bake within 50–60 minutes then serve.

Nutrition:
- Calories: 359
- Carbs: 45g
- Fat: 19g
- Protein: 4g

96. Quinoa, Corn, And Bean Salad

Preparation Time: 30 minutes
Cooking Time: 15 minutes
Servings: 6-8
Ingredients:

- 1 cup quinoa, rinsed and drained
- 2 cups water
- 1 (15-ounce) can corn, rinsed and drained
- 1 (15-ounce) can black beans
- 1 small zucchini, cubed
- 1/2 English cucumber, cubed
- 1/2 red bell pepper, diced
- 1 cup cherry tomatoes
- 1/4 cup finely chopped fresh cilantro
- 1/2 cup Quinoa Salad Dressing
- 1/4 teaspoon salt
- 1/4 teaspoon ground black pepper

Directions:

Put the quinoa and water and heat on medium-high setting. Boil. Decrease heat to low and simmer for about 15 minutes. Fluff with a fork and set aside.

Mix the corn, beans, zucchini, cucumber, bell pepper, tomatoes, and cilantro.

Once it cooled, add it to the vegetables and stir to combine. Add the dressing and stir to coat. Add the salt and pepper and toss. Serve.

Nutrition:

- Calories: 195.4
- Total Carbohydrate: 29.2 g
- Protein: 7.2 g
- Dietary Fiber: 6.3 g

97. Beet And Goat Cheese Salad

Preparation Time: 30 minutes
Cooking Time: 2 hours
Servings: 6
Ingredients:

- 4 medium beets
- 1/2 cup extra-virgin olive oil
- Juice of 1 lemon
- 1 teaspoon coconut sugar
- 1/2 teaspoon Dijon mustard
- 1/2 teaspoon salt
- 1/4 teaspoon ground black pepper
- 1 (12-ounce) bag spring mix salad greens
- 3 ounces goat cheese

Directions:

Slice the greens off the beets, leaving about 1" of the greens intact. Snip the root, leaving about 1" on the beet. Leave the skin on. Boil the beets in a medium saucepan over medium-high heat for 30–45 minutes or until fork tender.

In a bowl, whisk together the oil, lemon juice, coconut sugar, mustard, salt, and pepper for the salad dressing.

When done, carefully remove them from the hot water and peel them under cold running water. Let it cool then chop them into a medium dice.

For individual servings, place a handful of salad greens on each plate. Drizzle with the dressing and then top with diced beets and crumbled goat cheese.

Nutrition:

- Calories: 290.5
- Total Fat: 18.3 g
- Sodium: 466.6 mg
- Total Carbohydrate: 22.8 g

98. Cauli-Slaw

Preparation Time: 15 minutes
Cooking Time: 0 minutes
Servings: 6
Ingredients:

- 3 tablespoons gluten-free rice vinegar
- 1 tablespoon apple cider vinegar
- 2 teaspoons coconut sugar
- 1/3 cup mayonnaise
- 1/4 teaspoon salt
- 1/4 teaspoon ground black pepper
- 1/2 head cauliflower, sliced very thin
- 1 small stalk celery, minced
- 1/2 cup shredded carrots
- 1/8 cup red onion, minced
- 1/4 cup yellow bell pepper, minced

Directions:

Mix the vinegars, coconut sugar, mayonnaise, salt, and pepper to make the dressing in a mixing bowl.

Put the vegetables in a large bowl, followed with dressing, and toss.

Nutrition:

- 204. Cal.
- 6g. Carbs.
- 18g. Fat.
- 3g. Protein

99. Tabbouleh

Preparation Time: 15 minutes
Cooking Time: 0 minutes
Servings: 12
Ingredients:

- 1 bunch green onions
- ½ cup fresh mint leaves
- 1 cup flat leaf parsley
- 1 cucumber
- 2 cups cherry tomatoes
- 1 jicama
- ½ tsp. sea salt
- dash black pepper
- juice from ½ lemon
- 2 Tbsp. olive oil
- 2 cloves garlic, minced

Directions:

Peel the jicama and cut into 1-inch pieces. Put to a food processor to finely shredded. Put the shredded jicama in a separate bowl.

Slice the green onions, mint, parsley, cucumber, and cherry tomatoes. Put to the bowl.

Put the lemon juice, olive oil, sea salt, pepper, and garlic in a bowl. Mix well, and then put on top of the salad. Serve chilled. Enjoy!

Nutrition:

- Calories: 36
- Carbs: 8g
- Fat: 1g
- Protein: 2g

100. Mint Cabbage Salad

Preparation Time: 5 minutes
Cooking Time: 0 minutes
Servings: 6
Ingredients:

- 1 head green cabbage
- 2 Tbsp. dried mint
- juice from 1 lemon
- 4 garlic cloves, minced
- 1 tsp. olive oil
- pinch of sea salt

Directions:

Chop the cabbage very thinly and place in a deep bowl.

Combine the mint, lemon, garlic, and olive oil in a small bowl. Mix well.

Pour the mint dressing over the sliced cabbage. Add sea salt to taste. Enjoy!

Nutrition:

- Calories: 137
- Carbs: 11g
- Fat: 10g
- Protein: 2g

CHAPTER 7:

Second Courses With Side Dish

101. Peppered Broccoli Chicken

Preparation Time: 20 minutes
Cooking Time: 30 minutes
Servings: 4
Ingredients:

- 1 tbsp. sage (sliced)
- 1 cup broccoli florets
- 1 lb. (no bones and skin) chicken breast
- 3 pieces garlic cloves
- 1 cup tomato passata

What you'll need from the store cupboard:

- Salt and black pepper to taste
- 2 tbsp. olive oil

Directions:

1. Put the instant pot on the Sauté option, then put the oil and cook it. After that, put the chicken and garlic then heats it for 5 minutes.
2. Put the other ingredients, then cover it and heat it for 25 minutes at a high temperature.
3. Release the pressure gradually for 10 minutes then split them among your plates before eating.

Nutrition:

- **Calories:** 217
- **Carbs:** 5.9g
- **Protein:** 25.4g
- **Fat:** 10.1g
- **Fiber:** 1.8g

102. Buttery Cod

Preparation Time: 13 minutes
Cooking Time: 0 minutes
Servings: 2
Ingredients:

- 2 4-oz.cod fillets
- ½ medium lemon, sliced
- 2 tbsp. salted butter, melted.
- 1 tsp. old bay seasoning

Directions:

1. Place cod fillets into a 6-inch round baking dish. Brush each fillet with butter and sprinkle with old bay seasoning. Lay 2 lemon slices on each fillet
2. Cover the dish with foil and place it into the air fryer basket. Adjust the temperature to 350° F and set the timer for 8 minutes
3. Flip halfway through the cooking time.

4. When cooked, the internal temperature should be at least 145° F. Serve warm.

Nutrition:
- **Calories:** 179
- **Carbs:** 0 g
- **Protein:** 14 g
- **Fat:** 11 g
- **Fiber:** 0 g

103. Lime Baked Salmon

Preparation Time: 22 minutes
Cooking Time: 0
Servings: 2
Ingredients:

- 2 3-oz. salmon fillets, skin removed
- ¼ cup sliced pickled jalapeños
- ½ medium lime, juiced
- 2 tbsp. chopped cilantro
- 1 tbsp. salted butter; melted.
- ½ tsp. finely minced garlic
- 1 tsp. chili powder

Directions:
1. Place salmon fillets into a 6-inch round baking pan. Brush each with butter and sprinkle with chili powder and garlic
2. Place jalapeño slices on top and around salmon. Pour half of the lime juice over the salmon and cover with foil. Place pan into the air fryer basket. Adjust the temperature to 370° F and set the timer for 12 minutes
3. When fully cooked, salmon should flake easily with a fork and reach an internal temperature of at least 145° F.
4. To serve, spritz with remaining lime juice and garnish with cilantro.

Nutrition:
- **Calories:** 167 **Carbs:** 6 g
- **Protein:** 18 g **Fat:** 9 g
- **Fiber:** 7 g

104. Turkey Coriander Dish

Preparation Time: 20 minutes
Cooking Time: 20 minutes
Servings: 4
Ingredients:

- ½ bunch coriander (sliced)
- 1 cup chard (sliced)
- 1 piece (no bones and skin) turkey breast
- 1 and a half cup coconut cream
- 2 pieces garlic cloves

What you'll need from the store cupboard:

- 1 tbsp. melted ghee

Directions:
1. Put the instant pot on the Sauté option, then put the ghee and cook it. After that, put the garlic and meat then heat it for 5 minutes.
2. Put the other ingredients, then cover it and heat it for 25 minutes at a high temperature.
3. Release the pressure gradually for 10 minutes then split them among your plates before eating.

Nutrition:
- **Calories:** 225
- **Carbs:** 0.8 g
- **Protein:** 33.5 g **Fat:** 8.9 g
- **Fiber:** 0.2 g

105. Flank Steak Beef

Preparation Time: 10 minutes
Cooking Time: 20 minutes
Servings: 4
Ingredients:

- 1 lb. flank steaks, sliced
- ¼ cup xanthan gum
- 2 tsp. vegetable oil
- ½ tsp. ginger
- ½ cup soy sauce
- 1 tbsp. garlic, minced
- ½ cup water
- ¾ cup swerve, packed

Directions:

1. Preheat the Air fryer to 390° F and grease an Air fryer basket.
2. Coat the steaks with xanthan gum on both sides and transfer them into the Air fryer basket.
3. Cook for about 10 minutes and dish it out on a platter.
4. Meanwhile, cook the rest of the ingredients for the sauce in a saucepan.
5. Bring to a boil and pour over the steak slices to serve.

Nutrition:

- **Calories:** 372
- **Carbs:** 1.8 g
- **Protein:** 34 g
- **Fat:** 11.8 g
- **Sodium:** 871 mg

106. Sage Beef

Preparation Time: 10 minutes
Cooking Time: 30 minutes
Servings: 4
Ingredients:

- 2 lb. beef stew meat, cubed
- 1 tbsp. sage, chopped
- 2 tbsp. butter, melted
- ½ tsp. coriander, ground
- ½ tbsp. garlic powder
- 1 tsp. Italian seasoning
- Salt and black pepper to the taste

Directions:

1. In the air fryer's pan, mix the beef with the sage, melted butter, and the other ingredients, introduce the pan to the fryer and cook at 360° F for 30 minutes.
2. Divide everything between plates and serve.

Nutrition:

- **Calories:** 290
- **Carbs:** 20 g
- **Protein:** 29 g
- **Fat:** 11 g
- **Fiber:** 6 g

107. Roasted Tomato Brussels Sprouts

Preparation Time: 15 minutes
Cooking Time: 20 minutes
Servings: 4
Ingredients:

- 1 lb. (454 g) Brussels sprouts
- 1 tbsp. extra-virgin olive oil
- ½ cup sun-dried tomatoes
- 2 tbsp. lemon juice
- 1 tsp. lemon zest
- Salt and pepper, to taste

Directions:

1. Set oven 205° C. Prep large baking sheet with aluminum foil.
2. Toss the Brussels sprouts in the olive oil in a large bowl

until well coated. Sprinkle with salt and pepper.
3. Spread out the seasoned Brussels sprouts on the prepared baking sheet in a single layer.
4. Roast for 20 minutes, shaking halfway through.
5. Remove from the oven then situate in a bowl. Whisk tomatoes, lemon juice, and lemon zest, to incorporate. Serve immediately.

Nutrition:
- **Calories:** 111
- **Carbs:** 13.7 g
- **Fiber:** 4.9 g

108. Simple Sautéed Greens

Preparation Time: 10 minutes
Cooking Time: 10 minutes
Servings: 4
Ingredients:
- 2 tbsp. extra-virgin olive oil
- 1 lb. (454 g) Swiss chard
- 1 lb. (454 g) kale
- ½ tsp. ground cardamom
- 1 tbsp. lemon juice

Directions:
1. Heat up olive oil in a big skillet over medium-high heat.
2. Stir in Swiss chard, kale, cardamom, lemon juice to the skillet, and stir to combine. Cook for about 10 minutes, stirring continuously, or until the greens are wilted.
3. Sprinkle with salt and pepper and stir well.
4. Serve the greens on a plate while warm.

Nutrition:
- **Calories:** 139
- **Carbs:** 15.8 g
- **Fiber:** 3.9 g

109. Garlicky Mushrooms

Preparation Time: 10 minutes
Cooking Time: 12 minutes
Servings: 4
Ingredients:
- 1 tbsp. butter
- 2 tsp. extra-virgin olive oil
- 2 lb. button mushrooms
- 2 tsp. minced fresh garlic
- 1 tsp. chopped fresh thyme

Directions:
1. Heat up butter and olive oil in a huge skillet over medium-high heat.
2. Add the mushrooms and sauté for 10 minutes, stirring occasionally.
3. Stir in the garlic and thyme and cook for an additional 2 minutes.
4. Season and serve on a plate.

Nutrition:
- **Calories:** 96
- **Carbs:** 8.2 g
- **Fiber:** 1.7 g

110. Green Beans in Oven

Preparation Time: 5 minutes
Cooking Time: 17 minutes
Servings: 3
Ingredients:
- 12 oz. green bean pods
- 1 tbsp. olive oil
- ½ tsp. onion powder

- ⅛ tsp. pepper
- ⅛ tsp. salt

Directions:
1. Preheat oven to 350° F. Mix green beans with onion powder, salt, pepper, and oil.
2. Spread the seeds on the baking sheet.
3. Bake for 17 minutes or until you have a delicious aroma in the kitchen.

Nutrition:
- **Calories:** 37
- **Carbs:** 5.5 g
- **Protein:** 1.4 g

111. Parmesan Broiled Flounder

Preparation Time: 10 minutes
Cooking Time: 7 minutes
Servings: 2
Ingredients:

- 2 (4-oz) flounder
- 1,5 tbsp. Parmesan cheese
- 1,5 tbsp. mayonnaise
- ⅛ tsp. soy sauce
- ¼ tsp. chili sauce
- ⅛ tsp. salt-free lemon-pepper seasoning
- Salt and pepper, to taste

Directions:
1. Preheat flounder.
2. Mix cheese, reduced-fat mayonnaise, soy sauce, chili sauce, seasoning.
3. Put fish on a baking sheet coated with cooking spray, sprinkle with salt and pepper.
4. Spread Parmesan mixture over flounder.
5. Broil for 6 to 8 minutes or until a crust appears on the fish.

Nutrition:
- **Calories:** 200
- **Carbs:** 7 g
- **Fat:** 17 g

112. Wild Rice Salad With Cranberries and Almonds

Preparation Time: 6 minutes
Cooking Time: 25 minutes
Servings: 18
Ingredients:
Rice:

- 2 cups wild rice blend, rinsed
- 1 tsp. kosher salt
- 2 ½ cups vegetable broth

Dressing:

- ¼ cup extra-virgin olive oil
- ¼ cup white wine vinegar
- 1 ½ tsp. grated orange zest
- Juice of 1 medium orange (about ¼ cup)
- 1 tsp. honey or pure maple syrup

Salad:

- ¾ cup unsweetened dried cranberries
- ½ cup sliced almonds, toasted
- Freshly ground black pepper

Directions:
To make the rice:
1. In the electric pressure cooker, combine the rice, salt, and broth.
2. Close and lock the lid. Set the valve to sealing.

3. Cook on high pressure for 25 minutes.
4. When the cooking is complete, hit Cancel and allow the pressure to release naturally for 1 minutes, then quick release any remaining pressure.
5. Once the pin drops, unlock and remove the lid.
6. Let the rice cool briefly, then fluff it with a fork.

To make the dressing:
1. While the rice cooks, make the dressing: In a small jar with a screw-top lid, combine the olive oil, vinegar, zest, juice, and honey. (If you don't have a jar, whisk the ingredients together in a small bowl.) Shake to combine.

To make the salad:
1. Mix rice, cranberries, and almonds.
2. Add the dressing and season with pepper.
3. Serve warm or refrigerate.

Nutrition:
- **Calories:** 126
- **Carbs:** 18 g
- **Fiber:** 2 g

113. Low Fat Roasties

Preparation Time: 8 minutes
Cooking Time: 25 minutes
Servings: 2
Ingredients:
- 1 lb. roasting potatoes
- 1 garlic clove
- 1 cup vegetable stock
- 2 tbsp. olive oil

Directions:
1. Position potatoes in the steamer basket and add the stock into the Instant Pot.
2. Steam the potatoes in your Instant Pot for 15 minutes.
3. Depressurize and pour away the remaining stock.
4. Set to sauté and add the oil, garlic, and potatoes. Cook until brown.

Nutrition:
- **Calories:** 201
- **Carbs:** 3 g
- **Fat:** 6 g

114. Roasted Parsnips

Preparation Time: 9 minutes
Cooking Time: 25 minutes
Servings: 2
Ingredients:
- 1 lb. parsnips
- 1 cup vegetable stock
- 2 tbsp. herbs
- 2 tbsp. olive oil

Directions:
1. Put the parsnips in the steamer basket and add the stock into the Instant Pot.
2. Steam the parsnips in your Instant Pot for 15 minutes.
3. Depressurize and pour away the remaining stock.
4. Set to sauté and add the oil, herbs, and parsnips.
5. Cook until golden and crisp.

Nutrition:
- **Calories:** 130
- **Carbs:** 14 g
- **Protein:** 4 g

115. Beef, Olives, and Tomatoes

Preparation Time: 10 minutes
Cooking Time: 35 minutes
Servings: 4
Ingredients:

- 2 lb. beef stew meat, cubed
- 1 cup black olives, pitted and halved
- 1 cup cherry tomatoes, halved
- 1 tbsp. smoked paprika
- 3 tbsp. olive oil
- 1 tsp. coriander, ground
- Salt and black pepper to the taste

Directions:

1. In the air fryer's pan, mix the beef with the olives and the other ingredients, toss and cook at 390° F for 35 minutes.
2. Divide between plates and serve.

Nutrition:

- **Calories:** 291 **Carbs:** 20 g
- **Protein:** 26 g **Fat:** 12 g
- **Fiber:** 9 g

116. Easy Lime Lamb Cutlets

Preparation Time: 4 hours 20 minutes
Cooking Time: 8 minutes
Servings: 4
Ingredients:

- ¼ cup freshly squeezed lime juice - 2 tbsp. lime zest
- 2 tbsp. chopped fresh parsley
- Sea salt and freshly ground black pepper, to taste
- 1 tbsp. extra-virgin olive oil
- 12 lamb cutlets (about 1½ lb. / 680 g in total)

Directions:

1. Combine the lime juice and zest, parsley, salt, black pepper, and olive oil in a large bowl. Stir to mix well.
2. Dunk the lamb cutlets in the bowl of the lime mixture, then toss to coat well. Wrap the bowl in plastic and refrigerate to marinate for at least 4 hours.
3. Preheat the oven to 450° F (235° C) or broil. Line a baking sheet with aluminum foil.
4. Remove the bowl from the refrigerator and let sit for 10 minutes, then discard the marinade. Arrange the lamb cutlets on the baking sheet.
5. Broil the lamb in the preheated oven for 8 minutes or until it reaches your desired doneness. Flip the cutlets with tongs to make sure they are cooked evenly.
6. Serve immediately.

Tip: If you are fancy about the spicy taste of the lamb cutlets, you can sprinkle the cooked cutlets with chipotle chili powder or red pepper flakes before serving.

Nutrition:

- **Calories:** 297
- **Carbs:** 1.0 g
- **Protein:** 31.0 g
- **Fat:** 18.8 g
- **Fiber:** 0 g
- **Sodium:** 100 mg

117. Sumptuous Lamb and Pomegranate Salad

Preparation Time: 8 hours 35 minutes
Cooking Time: 30 minutes
Servings: 8
Ingredients:

- 1 ½ cups pomegranate juice
- 4 tbsp. olive oil, divided
- 1 tbsp. ground cinnamon
- 1 tsp. cumin
- 1 tbsp. ground ginger
- 3 cloves garlic, chopped
- Salt and freshly ground black pepper, to taste
- 1 (4-lb. / 1.8-kg) lamb leg, deboned, butterflied, and fat trimmed
- 2 tbsp. pomegranate balsamic vinegar
- 2 tsp. Dijon mustard
- ½ cup pomegranate seeds
- 5 cups baby kale
- 4 cups fresh green beans, blanched
- ¼ cup toasted walnut halves
- 2 fennel bulbs, thinly sliced
- 2 tbsp. Gorgonzola cheese

Directions:

1. Mix the pomegranate juice, 1 tbsp. of olive oil, cinnamon, cumin, ginger, garlic, salt, and black pepper in a large bowl. Stir to mix well.
2. Dunk the lamb leg in the mixture, press to coat well. Wrap the bowl in plastic and refrigerate to marinate for at least 8 hours.
3. Remove the bowl from the refrigerator and let sit for 20 minutes. Pat the lamb dry with paper towels.
4. Preheat the grill to high heat.
5. Brush the grill grates with 1 tbsp. of olive oil, then arrange the lamb on the grill grates.
6. Grill for 30 minutes or until the internal temperature of the lamb reaches at least 145° F (63° C). Flip the lamb halfway through the cooking time.
7. Remove the lamb from the grill and wrap it with aluminum foil. Let stand for 15 minutes.
8. Meanwhile, combine the vinegar, mustard, salt, black pepper, and remaining olive oil in a separate large bowl. Stir to mix well.
9. Add the remaining ingredients and lamb leg to the bowl and toss to combine well. Serve immediately.

Tips: You can use the same amount of sliced red grapes to replace the pomegranate seeds. If you don't have pomegranate balsamic vinegar, you can juice use the balsamic vinegar to replace it.

Nutrition:

- **Calories:** 380
- **Carbs:** 16.0 g
- **Protein:** 32.0 g
- **Fat:** 21.0 g
- **Fiber:** 5.0 g
- **Sodium:** 240 mg

118. Pork Spare Ribs

Preparation Time: 15 minutes
Cooking Time: 20 minutes
Servings: 6
Ingredients:

- 5 to 6 garlic cloves, minced
- ½ cup rice vinegar
- 2 tbsp. soy sauce
- Salt and ground black pepper, as required
- 12 1-inch pork spare ribs
- ½ cup cornstarch
- 2 tbsp. olive oil

Directions:

1. In a large bowl, mix together the garlic, vinegar, soy sauce, salt, and black pepper.
2. Add the ribs and generously coat with the mixture.
3. Refrigerate to marinate overnight.
4. In a shallow bowl, place the cornstarch.
5. Coat the ribs evenly with cornstarch and then, drizzle with oil.
6. Set the temperature of the air fryer to 390° F. Grease an air fryer basket.
7. Arrange ribs into the prepared air fryer basket in a single layer.
8. Air fry for about 10 minutes per side.
9. Remove from air fryer and transfer the ribs onto serving plates.
10. Serve immediately.

Nutrition:

- **Calories:** 557 **Carbs:** 11 g
- **Protein:** 35 g
- **Fat:** 51.3 g
- **Sodium:** 997 mg

119. Lime Trout and Shallots

Preparation Time: 17 minutes
Cooking Time: 0
Servings: 4
Ingredients:

- 4 trout fillets, boneless
- 3 garlic cloves, minced
- 6 shallots, chopped
- ½ cup butter, melted
- ½ cup olive oil
- Juice of 1 lime
- A pinch of salt and black pepper

Directions:

1. In a pan that fits the air fryer, combine the fish with the shallots and the rest of the ingredients, toss gently
2. Put the pan in the machine and cook at 390° F for 12 minutes, flipping the fish halfway.
3. Divide between plates and serve with a side salad.

Nutrition:

- **Calories:** 270
- **Carbs:** 6 g
- **Protein:** 12 g
- **Fat:** 12 g
- **Fiber:** 4 g

120. Fish and Salsa

Preparation Time: 20 minutes
Cooking Time: 0
Servings: 4
Ingredients:

- 4 sea bass fillets, boneless
- 3 garlic cloves, minced
- 3 tomatoes, roughly chopped.
- 2 spring onions, chopped.

- ¼ cup chicken stock
- 1 tbsp. balsamic vinegar
- 1 tbsp. olive oil
- A pinch of salt and black pepper

Directions:
1. In a blender, combine all the ingredients except the fish and pulse well.
2. Put the mix in a pan that fits the air fryer, add the fish, toss gently, introduce the pan in the fryer and cook at 380° F for 15 minutes. Divide between plates and serve.

Nutrition:
- **Calories:** 261
- **Carbs:** 7 g
- **Protein:** 11 g
- **Fat:** 11 g
- **Fiber:** 4 g

121. Crab Legs

Preparation Time: 20 minutes
Cooking Time: 0 minutes
Servings: 4
Ingredients:

- 3 lb. crab legs
- ¼ cup salted butter; melted and divided
- Juice of ½ medium lemon
- ¼ tsp. garlic powder

Directions:
1. Take a large bowl, drizzle 2 tbsp. of butter over crab legs. Place crab legs into the air fryer basket.
2. Adjust the temperature to 400° F and set the timer for 15 minutes. Shake the air fryer basket to toss the crab legs halfway through the cooking time
3. In a small bowl, mix remaining butter, garlic powder, and lemon juice
4. To serve, crack open crab legs and remove meat. Dip in lemon butter.

Nutrition:
- **Calories:** 123
- **Carbs:** 4 g
- **Protein:** 17 g
- **Fat:** 6 g
- **Fiber:** 0 g

122. Teriyaki Chicken and Broccoli

Preparation Time: 5 minutes
Cooking Time: 20 minutes
Servings: 4
Ingredients:
Sauce:

- ½ cup water
- 2 tbsp. low-sodium soy sauce
- 2 tbsp. honey
- 1 tbsp. rice vinegar
- ¼ tsp. garlic powder
- Pinch ground ginger
- 1 tbsp. cornstarch

Entrée:

- 1 tbsp. sesame oil
- 4 (4-oz. / 113-g) boneless, skinless chicken breasts, cut into bite-size cubes
- 1 (12-oz. / 340-g) bag frozen broccoli
- 1 (12-oz. / 340-g) bag frozen cauliflower rice

Directions:
Make the sauce:
1. In a small saucepan, whisk together the water, soy sauce, honey, rice vinegar, garlic powder, and ginger. Add the cornstarch and whisk until it is fully incorporated.
2. Over medium heat, bring the teriyaki sauce to a boil. Let the sauce boil for 1 minute to thicken. Remove the sauce from the heat and set aside.

Make the entrée:
1. Heat a large skillet over medium-low heat. When hot, add the oil and the chicken. Cook for 5 to 7 minutes, until the chicken, is cooked through, stirring as needed. Steam the broccoli and cauliflower rice in the microwave according to the package directions.
2. Divide the cauliflower rice into four equal portions. Put one-quarter of the broccoli and chicken over each portion and top with the teriyaki sauce.

Nutrition:
- **Calories:** 247 **Carbs:** 20 g
- **Protein:** 29 g **Fat:** 7 g
- **Fiber:** 5 g **Sodium:** 418 mg

123. Coconut Lime Chicken

Preparation Time: 5 minutes
Cooking Time: 15 minutes
Servings: 4
Ingredients:
- 1 tbsp. coconut oil
- 4 (4-oz. / 113-g) boneless, skinless chicken breasts
- ½ tsp. salt
- 1 red bell pepper, cut into ¼-inch-thick slices
- 16 asparagus spears, bottom ends trimmed
- 1 cup unsweetened coconut milk
- 2 tbsp. freshly squeezed lime juice
- ½ tsp. garlic powder
- ¼ tsp. red pepper flakes
- ¼ cup chopped fresh cilantro

Directions:
1. In a large skillet, heat the oil over medium-low heat. When hot, add the chicken.
2. Season the chicken with salt. Cook for 5 minutes, then flip.
3. Push the chicken to the side of the skillet, and add the bell pepper and asparagus. Cook, covered, for 5 minutes.
4. Meanwhile, in a small bowl, whisk together the coconut milk, lime juice, garlic powder, and red pepper flakes.
5. Add the coconut milk mixture to the skillet, and boil over high heat for 2 to 3 minutes.
6. Top with the cilantro.

Nutrition:
- **Calories:** 321
- **Carbs:** 11 g
- **Protein:** 30 g
- **Fat:** 19 g
- **Fiber:** 4 g
- **Sodium:** 378 mg

124. Roasted Vegetable and Chicken Salad

Preparation Time: 10 minutes
Cooking Time: 10 to 13 minutes
Servings: 4
Ingredients:

- 3 boneless, skinless chicken breasts, cut into 1-inch cubes
- 1 small red onion, sliced
- 1 orange bell pepper, sliced
- 1 cup sliced yellow summer squash
- 4 tbsp. honey mustard salad dressing, divided
- ½ tsp. dried thyme
- ½ cup mayonnaise
- 2 tbsp. freshly squeezed lemon juice

Directions:

1. Place the chicken, onion, pepper, and squash in the air fryer basket. Drizzle with 1 tbsp. of the honey mustard salad dressing, add the thyme, and toss.
2. Roast at 400° F (204° C) for 10 to 13 minutes or until the chicken is 165° F (74° C) on a food thermometer, tossing the food once during cooking time.
3. Transfer the chicken and vegetables to a bowl and mix in the remaining 3 tbsp. of honey mustard salad dressing, mayonnaise, and lemon juice. Serve on lettuce leaves, if desired.

Nutrition:

- **Calories:** 495 **Carbs:** 18 g
- **Protein:** 51 g **Fat:** 23 g
- **Fiber:** 2 g **Sodium:** 439 mg

125. Chicken Satay

Preparation Time: 12 minutes
Cooking Time: 12 to 18 minutes
Servings: 4
Ingredients:

- ½ cup crunchy peanut butter
- ⅓ cup chicken broth
- 3 tbsp. low-sodium soy sauce
- 2 tbsp. freshly squeezed lemon juice
- 2 cloves garlic, minced
- 2 tbsp. olive oil
- 1 tsp. curry powder
- 1 lb. (454 g) chicken tenders

Directions:

1. In a medium bowl, combine the peanut butter, chicken broth, soy sauce, lemon juice, garlic, olive oil, and curry powder, and mix well with a wire whisk until smooth. Remove 2 tbsp. of this mixture to a small bowl. Put the remaining sauce into a serving bowl and set aside.
2. Add the chicken tenders to the bowl with the 2 tbsp. of sauce and stir to coat. Let stand for a few minutes to marinate, and then run a bamboo skewer through each chicken tender lengthwise.
3. Put the chicken in the air fryer basket and air fry in batches at 390° F (199° C) for 6 to 9 minutes or until the chicken reaches 165° F (74° C) on a meat thermometer.

4. Serve the chicken with the reserved sauce.

Nutrition:
- **Calories:** 449
- **Carbs:** 8 g
- **Protein:** 46 g
- **Fat:** 28 g
- **Fiber:** 2 g
- **Sodium:** 984 mg

126. Chicken Fajitas With Avocados

Preparation Time: 10 minutes
Cooking Time: 10 to 14 minutes
Servings: 4
Ingredients:

- 4 boneless, skinless chicken breasts, sliced
- 1 small red onion, sliced
- 2 red bell peppers, sliced
- ½ cup spicy ranch salad dressing, divided
- ½ tsp. dried oregano
- 8 corn tortillas
- 2 cups torn butter lettuce
- 2 avocados, peeled and chopped

Directions:

1. Place the chicken, onion, and pepper in the air fryer basket. Drizzle with 1 tbsp. of the salad dressing and add the oregano. Toss to combine.
2. Air fry at 380° F (193° C) for 10 to 14 minutes or until the chicken is 165° F (74° C) on a food thermometer.
3. Transfer the chicken and vegetables to a bowl and toss with the remaining salad dressing.
4. Serve the chicken mixture with the tortillas, lettuce, and avocados, and let everyone make their own creations.

Nutrition:
- **Calories:** 784
- **Carbs:** 39 g
- **Protein:** 72 g
- **Fat:** 38 g
- **Fiber:** 12 g
- **Sodium:** 397 mg

127. Crispy Buttermilk Fried Chicken

Preparation Time: 7 minutes
Cooking Time: 20 to 25 minutes
Servings: 4
Ingredients:

- 6 chicken pieces: drumsticks, breasts, and thighs
- 1 cup flour
- 2 tsp. paprika
- Pinch salt
- Freshly ground black pepper, to taste
- $1/3$ cup buttermilk
- 2 eggs
- 2 tbsp. olive oil
- 1 ½ cups bread crumbs

Directions:

1. Pat the chicken dry. In a shallow bowl, combine the flour, paprika, salt, and pepper.
2. In another bowl, beat the buttermilk with the eggs until smooth.
3. In a third bowl, combine the olive oil and bread crumbs until mixed.
4. Dredge the chicken in the flour, then into the eggs to

coat, and finally into the bread crumbs, patting the crumbs firmly onto the chicken skin.
5. Air fry the chicken at 370° F (188° C) for 20 to 25 minutes, turning each piece over halfway during cooking until the meat registers 165° F (74° C) on a meat thermometer and the chicken is brown and crisp. Let cool for 5 minutes, then serve.

Nutrition:
- **Calories:** 645
- **Carbs:** 55 g
- **Protein:** 62 g
- **Fat:** 17 g
- **Fiber:** 3 g
- **Sodium:** 495 mg

128. Garlicky Chicken With Creamer Potatoes

Preparation Time: 10 minutes
Cooking Time: 25 minutes
Servings: 4
Ingredients:

- 1 (2 ½ to 3-lb. / 1.1- to 1.4-kg) broiler-fryer whole chicken
- 2 tbsp. olive oil
- ½ tsp. garlic salt
- 8 cloves garlic, peeled
- 1 slice lemon
- ½ tsp. dried thyme
- ½ tsp. dried marjoram
- 12 to 16 creamer potatoes, scrubbed

Directions:
1. Do not wash the chicken before cooking. Remove it from its packaging and pat the chicken dry.
2. Combine the olive oil and salt in a small bowl. Rub half of this mixture on the inside of the chicken, under the skin, and on the chicken skin. Place the garlic cloves and lemon slice inside the chicken. Sprinkle the chicken with thyme and marjoram.
3. Put the chicken in the air fryer basket. Surround with the potatoes and drizzle the potatoes with the remaining olive oil mixture.
4. Roast at 380° F (193° C) for 25 minutes, then test the temperature of the chicken. It should be 160° F (71° C). Test at the thickest part of the breast, making sure the probe doesn't touch bone. If the chicken isn't done yet, return it to the air fryer and roast it for 4 to 5 minutes, or until the temperature is 160° F (71° C).
5. When the chicken is done, transfer it and the potatoes to a serving platter and cover with foil. Let the chicken rest for 5 minutes before serving.

Nutrition:
- **Calories:** 492
- **Carbs:** 20 g
- **Protein:** 68 g
- **Fat:** 14 g
- **Fiber:** 3 g
- **Sodium:** 151 mg

129. Honey Lemon Garlic Chicken

Preparation Time: 10 minutes
Cooking Time: 16 to 19 minutes
Servings: 4
Ingredients:

- 4 (5-oz. / 142-g) low-sodium boneless, skinless chicken breasts, cut into 4- by ½-inch strips
- 2 tsp. olive oil
- 2 tbsp. cornstarch
- 3 garlic cloves, minced
- ½ cup low-sodium chicken broth
- ¼ cup freshly squeezed lemon juice
- 1 tbsp. honey
- ½ tsp. dried thyme
- Brown rice, cooked (optional)

Directions:

1. In a large bowl, mix the chicken and olive oil. Sprinkle with the cornstarch. Toss to coat.
2. Add the garlic and transfer to a baking pan. Bake in the air fryer at 400° F (204° C) for 10 minutes, stirring once during cooking.
3. Add the chicken broth, lemon juice, honey, and thyme to the chicken mixture. Bake for 6 to 9 minutes more, or until the sauce is slightly thickened and the chicken reaches an internal temperature of 165° F (74° C) on a meat thermometer. Serve over hot cooked brown rice, if desired.

Nutrition:

- **Calories:** 214
- **Fat:** 4 g
- **Protein:** 33 g
- **Carbs:** 10 g
- **Fiber:** 0 g
- **Sodium:** 100 mg

130. Baked Lemon Pepper Chicken Drumsticks

Preparation Time: 5 minutes
Cooking Time: 22 minutes
Servings: 6 drumsticks
Ingredients:

- Olive oil spray
- 6 chicken drumsticks
- 1 tsp. lemon pepper
- ½ tsp. salt
- ½ tsp. granulated garlic
- ½ tsp. onion powder

Directions:

1. Spray the chicken with olive oil and spray the air fryer basket or line it with parchment paper.
2. In a small bowl, combine the lemon pepper, salt, garlic, and onion powder.
3. Place the chicken in the prepared air fryer basket and sprinkle with half of the seasoning mixture.
4. Bake at 370° F (188° C) for 10 minutes.
5. Flip the drumsticks and spray them with more olive oil and sprinkle with the remaining seasoning.
6. Place the chicken back in the air fryer, bake for an additional 12 minutes, and serve.

7. The chicken is done when the internal temperature reaches 180° F (82° C) and the juices run clear. It should look slightly crisp on the outside.

Nutrition:
- **Calories:** 195
- **Carbs:** 1 g
- **Protein:** 23 g
- **Fat:** 11 g
- **Fiber:** 0 g
- **Sodium:** 332 mg

131. Pork Chops With Grape Sauce

Preparation Time: 15 minutes
Cooking Time: 25 minutes
Servings: 4
Ingredients:
- Cooking spray
- 4 pork chops
- ¼ cup onion, sliced
- 1 clove garlic, minced
- ½ cup low-sodium chicken broth
- ¾ cup apple juice
- 1 tbsp. cornstarch
- 1 tbsp. balsamic vinegar
- 1 tsp. honey
- 1 cup seedless red grapes, sliced in half

Directions:
1. Spray oil on your pan. Put it over medium heat.
2. Add the pork chops to the pan. Cook for 5 minutes per side. Remove and set aside.
3. Add onion and garlic. Cook for 2 minutes.
4. Pour in the broth and apple juice. Bring to a boil.
5. Reduce heat to simmer. Put the pork chops back to the skillet.
6. Simmer for 4 minutes.
7. In a bowl, mix the cornstarch, vinegar, and honey. Add to the pan.
8. Cook until the sauce has thickened.
9. Add the grapes.
10. Pour sauce over the pork chops before serving.

Nutrition:
- **Calories:** 188
- **Total carbs:** 18 g
- **Protein:** 19 g
- **Total fat:** 4 g
- **Saturated fat:** 1 g
- **Cholesterol:** 47 mg
- **Sodium:** 117 mg
- **Dietary fiber:** 1 g
- **Potassium:** 759 mg

132. Roasted Pork & Apples

Preparation Time: 15 minutes
Cooking Time: 30 minutes
Servings: 4
Ingredients:
- Salt and pepper to taste
- ½ tsp. dried, crushed
- 1 lb. pork tenderloin
- 1 tbsp. canola oil
- 1 onion, sliced into wedges
- 3 cooking apples, sliced into wedges
- ⅔ cup apple cider
- Sprigs fresh sage

Directions:
1. In a bowl, mix salt, pepper, and sage. Season both sides of pork with this mixture.

2. Place a pan over medium heat. Brown both sides.
3. Transfer to a roasting pan.
4. Add the onion on top and around the pork.
5. Drizzle oil on top of the pork and apples.
6. Roast in the oven at 425° F for 10 minutes.
7. Add the apples, roast for another 15 minutes.
8. In a pan, boil the apple cider and then simmer for 10 minutes.
9. Pour the apple cider sauce over the pork before serving.

Nutrition:
- **Calories:** 239
- **Total carbs:** 22 g
- **Protein:** 24 g
- **Total fat:** 6 g
- **Saturated fat:** 1 g
- **Cholesterol:** 74 mg
- **Sodium:** 209 mg
- **Dietary fiber:** 3 g
- **Potassium:** 655 mg

133. Pork With Cranberry Relish

Preparation Time: 30 minutes
Cooking Time: 30 minutes
Servings: 4
Ingredients:
- 12 oz. pork tenderloin, fat trimmed and sliced crosswise
- Salt and pepper to taste
- ¼ cup all-purpose flour
- 2 tbsp. olive oil
- 1 onion, sliced thinly
- ¼ cup dried cranberries
- ¼ cup low-sodium chicken broth
- 1 tbsp. balsamic vinegar

Directions:
1. Flatten each slice of pork using a mallet.
2. In a dish, mix the salt, pepper, and flour.
3. Dip each pork slice into the flour mixture.
4. Add oil to a pan over medium-high heat.
5. Cook pork for 3 minutes per side or until golden crispy.
6. Transfer to a serving plate and cover with foil.
7. Cook the onion in the pan for 4 minutes.
8. Stir in the rest of the ingredients.
9. Simmer until the sauce has thickened.

Nutrition:
- **Calories:** 211
- **Total carbs:** 15 g
- **Protein:** 18 g
- **Total fat:** 9 g
- **Saturated fat:** 2 g
- **Cholesterol:** 53 mg
- **Sodium:** 116 mg
- **Dietary fiber:** 1 g
- **Potassium:** 378 mg

134. Shrimp & Veggies Curry

Preparation Time: 10 minutes
Cooking Time: 30 minutes
Servings: 6
Ingredients:
- 2 tsp. olive oil
- 1 ½ medium white onions, sliced
- 2 medium green bell peppers, seeded and sliced

- 3 medium carrots, peeled and sliced thinly
- 3 garlic cloves, chopped finely
- 1 tbsp. fresh ginger, chopped finely
- 2 ½ tsp. curry powder
- 1 ½ lb. shrimp, peeled and deveined
- 1 cup filtered water
- 2 tbsp. fresh lime juice
- Salt and ground black pepper, as required
- 2 tbsp. fresh cilantro, chopped

Directions:
1. In a large skillet, heat oil over medium-high heat and sauté the onion for about 4 to 5 minutes.
2. Add the bell peppers and carrot and sauté for about 3 to 4 minutes.
3. Add the garlic, ginger, and curry powder and sauté for about 1 minute.
4. Add the shrimp and sauté for about 1 minute.
5. Stir in the water and cook for about 4 to 6 minutes, stirring occasionally.
6. Stir in lime juice and remove from heat.
7. Serve hot with the garnishing of cilantro.

Meal prep tip: Transfer the curry into a large bowl and set it aside to cool. Divide the curry into 6 containers evenly. Cover the containers and refrigerate for 1 to 2 days. Reheat in the microwave before serving.

Nutrition:
- **Calories:** 193
- **Total carbs:** 12 g
- **Protein:** 27.1 g
- **Total fat:** 3.8 g
- **Saturated fat:** 0.9 g
- **Cholesterol:** 239 mg
- **Sugar:** 4.7 g
- **Fiber:** 2.3 g
- **Sodium:** 328 mg
- **Potassium:** 437 mg

135. Lemon and Honey Pork Tenderloin

Preparation Time: 5 minutes
Cooking Time: 10 minutes
Servings: 4
Ingredients:
- 1 (1-lb. / 454-g) pork tenderloin, cut into ½-inch slices
- 1 tbsp. olive oil
- 1 tbsp. freshly squeezed lemon juice
- 1 tbsp. honey
- ½ tsp. grated lemon zest
- ½ tsp. dried marjoram
- Pinch salt
- Freshly ground black pepper, to taste

Directions:
1. Put the pork tenderloin slices in a medium bowl.
2. In a minor bowl, combine the olive oil, lemon juice, honey, lemon zest, marjoram, salt, and pepper. Mix.
3. Pour this marinade over the tenderloin slices and massage gently with your hand to work it into the pork.

4. Place the pork in the air fryer basket and roast at 400° F (204° C) for 10 minutes or until the pork registers at least 145° F (63° C) using a meat thermometer.

Nutrition:
- **Calories:** 208
- **Carbs:** 5 g
- **Protein:** 30 g
- **Fat:** 8 g
- **Fiber:** 0 g
- **Sodium:** 104 mg

136. Dijon Pork Tenderloin

Preparation Time: 10 minutes
Cooking Time: 12 to 14 minutes
Servings: 4

Ingredients:
- 1 lb. (454 g) pork tenderloin, cut into 1-inch slices
- Pinch salt
- Freshly ground black pepper, to taste
- 2 tbsp. Dijon mustard
- 1 clove garlic, minced
- ½ tsp. dried basil
- 1 cup soft bread crumbs
- 2 tbsp. olive oil

Directions:
1. Slightly pound the pork slices until they are about ¾-inch thick. Sprinkle with salt and pepper on both sides.
2. Coat the pork with the Dijon mustard and sprinkle with the garlic and basil.
3. On a plate, combine the bread crumbs and olive oil and mix well. Coat the pork slices with the bread crumb mixture, patting, so the crumbs adhere.
4. Place the pork in the air fryer basket, leaving a little space between each piece. Air fry at 390° F (199° C) for 12 to 14 minutes or until the pork reaches at least 145 °F (63° C) on a meat thermometer and the coating is crisp and brown. Serve immediately.

Nutrition:
- **Calories:** 336
- **Carbs:** 20 g
- **Protein:** 34 g
- **Fat:** 13 g
- **Fiber:** 2 g
- **Sodium:** 390 mg

137. Air Fryer Pork Satay

Preparation Time: 15 minutes
Cooking Time: 9 to 14 minutes
Servings: 4

Ingredients:
- 1 (1-lb. / 454-g) pork tenderloin, cut into 1 ½-inch cubes
- ¼ cup minced onion
- 2 garlic cloves, minced
- 1 jalapeño pepper, minced
- 2 tbsp. freshly squeezed lime juice
- 2 tbsp. coconut milk
- 2 tbsp. unsalted peanut butter
- 2 tsp. curry powder

Directions:
1. In a medium bowl, mix the pork, onion, garlic, jalapeño, lime juice, coconut milk,

peanut butter, and curry powder until well combined. Let position for 10 minutes at room temperature.
2. With a slotted spoon, remove the pork from the marinade. Reserve the marinade.
3. Thread the pork onto about 8 bamboo or metal skewers. Air fry at 380° F (193° C) for 9 to 14 minutes, brushing once with the reserved marinade until the pork reaches at least 145° F (63° C) on a meat thermometer. Discard any remaining marinade. Serve immediately.

Nutrition:
- **Calories:** 195
- **Carbs:** 7 g
- **Protein:** 25 g
- **Fat:** 7 g
- **Fiber:** 1 g
- **Sodium:** 65 mg

138. Pork Burgers With Red Cabbage Slaw

Preparation Time: 20 minutes
Cooking Time: 7 to 9 minutes
Servings: 4
Ingredients:
- ½ cup Greek yogurt
- 2 tbsp. low-sodium mustard, divided
- 1 tbsp. freshly squeezed lemon juice
- ¼ cup sliced red cabbage
- ¼ cup grated carrots
- 1 lb. (454 g) lean ground pork
- ½ tsp. paprika
- 1 cup mixed baby lettuce greens
- 2 small tomatoes, sliced
- 8 small low-sodium whole-wheat sandwich buns, cut in half

Directions:
1. In a lesser bowl, syndicate the yogurt, 1 tbsp. of mustard, lemon juice, cabbage, and carrots; mix and refrigerate.
2. In a medium bowl, combine the pork, remaining 1 tbsp. of mustard, and paprika. Form into 8 small patties.
3. Lay the patties into the air fryer basket. Air fry at 400° F (204° C) for 7 to 9 minutes, or until the patties register 165° F (74° C) as tested with a meat thermometer.
4. Assemble the burgers by placing some of the lettuce greens on a bun bottom. Top with a tomato slice, the patties, and the cabbage mixture. Add the bun top and serve immediately.

Nutrition:
- **Calories:** 473 **Carbs:** 51 g
- **Protein:** 35 g
- **Fat:** 15 g
- **Fiber:** 8 g
- **Sodium:** 138mg

139. Balsamic-Glazed Chicken

Preparation Time: 5 minutes
Cooking Time: 22 minutes
Servings: 4
Ingredients:
Glaze:

- 1 tbsp. olive oil
- 2 tsp. balsamic vinegar
- 1 tsp. minced garlic
- 1 tsp. honey
- ½ tsp. cornstarch
- ¼ tsp. salt
- ¼ tsp. ground black pepper

Chicken:
- Olive oil spray
- 4 bone-in chicken thighs
- 2 tsp. granulated garlic, divided
- 1 tsp. salt, divided
- ½ tsp. ground black pepper, divided
- ¼ tsp. onion powder, divided

Directions:
Make the glaze:
1. In a small bowl, whisk together the olive oil, balsamic vinegar, garlic, honey, cornstarch, salt, and pepper. Set aside.

Make the chicken:
1. Spray the chicken and the air fryer basket with olive oil.
2. Place the chicken in the air fryer basket, and sprinkle with about half of the garlic, salt, pepper, and onion powder.
3. Bake at 380° F (193° C) for 10 minutes.
4. Remove the chicken and flip the pieces. Spray it with more olive oil, and sprinkle with the remaining seasoning.
5. Place the chicken back in the air fryer and bake for an additional 10 minutes.
6. Remove the chicken, and brush with the prepared glaze. Bake for an additional 2 minutes, or until the sauce is sticky and caramelized, and serve.

Nutrition:
- **Calories:** 263
- **Carbs:** 3 g
- **Protein:** 38 g
- **Fat:** 11 g
- **Fiber:** 0 g
- **Sodium:** 911 mg

140. Cajun Salmon

Preparation Time: 12 minutes
Cooking Time: 0 minutes
Servings: 2
Ingredients:
- 2 4-oz. salmon fillets, skin removed
- 2 tbsp. unsalted butter; melted.
- 1 tsp. paprika
- ¼ tsp. ground black pepper
- ⅛ tsp. ground cayenne pepper
- ½ tsp. garlic powder.

Directions:
1. Brush each fillet with butter. Combine remaining ingredients in a small bowl and then rub onto fish. Place fillets into the air fryer basket
2. Adjust the temperature to 390° F and set the timer for 7 minutes. When fully cooked, the internal temperature will be 145° F. Serve immediately.

Nutrition:
- **Calories:** 253 **Carbs:** 4 g
- **Protein:** 29 g **Fat:** 16 g
- **Fiber:** 4 g

141. Trout and Zucchinis

Preparation Time: 20 minutes
Cooking Time: 0
Servings: 4
Ingredients:

- 3 zucchinis, cut in medium chunks
- 4 trout fillets, boneless
- ¼ cup tomato sauce
- 1 garlic clove, minced
- ½ cup cilantro, chopped.
- 1 tbsp. lemon juice
- 2 tbsp. olive oil
- Salt and black pepper to taste.

Directions:

1. In a pan that fits your air fryer, mix the fish with the other ingredients, toss, introduce in the fryer and cook at 380° F for 15 minutes. Divide everything between plates and serve right away

Nutrition:

- **Calories:** 220
- **Carbs:** 6 g
- **Protein:** 9 g
- **Fat:** 12 g
- **Fiber:** 4 g

142. BBQ Pork Ribs

Preparation Time: 15 minutes
Cooking Time: 26 minutes
Servings: 4
Ingredients:

- ¼ cup honey, divided
- ¾ cup BBQ sauce
- 2 tbsp. tomato ketchup
- 1 tbsp. Worcestershire sauce*
- 1 tbsp. soy sauce
- ½ tsp. garlic powder
- Freshly ground white pepper, to taste
- 1 ¾ lb. pork ribs

Directions:

1. In a bowl, mix together 3 tbsp. of honey and the remaining ingredients except for pork ribs.
2. Add the pork ribs and generously coat with the mixture.
3. Refrigerate to marinate for about 20 minutes.
4. Set the temperature of the air fryer to 355° F. Grease an air fryer basket
5. Arrange ribs into the prepared air fryer basket in a single layer.
6. Air fry for about 13 minutes per side.
7. Remove from air fryer and transfer the ribs onto plates.
8. Drizzle with the remaining honey and serve immediately.

Note: (Worcestershire sauce*) The other ingredients that make up this savory sauce usually include onions, molasses, high fructose corn syrup (depending on the country of production), salt, garlic, tamarind, cloves, chili pepper extract, water, and natural flavorings.

Nutrition:

- **Calories:** 691
- **Carbs:** 37.7 g
- **Protein:** 53.1 g
- **Fat:** 31.3 g
- **Sodium:** 991 mg

143. Glazed Pork Shoulder

Preparation Time: 15 minutes
Cooking Time: 18 minutes
Servings: 5
Ingredients:

- ⅓ cup soy sauce
- 2 tbsp. maple sugar
- 1 tbsp. honey
- 2 lb. pork shoulder, cut into 1½-inch thick slices

Directions:

1. In a bowl, mix together all the soy sauce, maple sugar, and honey.
2. Add the pork and generously coat with marinade.
3. Cover and refrigerate to marinate for about 4 to 6 hours.
4. Set the temperature of the air fryer to 335° F. Grease an air fryer basket.
5. Place the pork shoulder into the prepared air fryer basket.
6. Air fry for about 10 minutes and then, another 6 to 8 minutes at 390° F.
7. Remove from air fryer and transfer the pork shoulder onto a platter.
8. With a piece of foil, cover the pork for about 10 minutes before serving.
9. Enjoy!

Nutrition:

- **Calories:** 475
- **Carbs:** 8 g
- **Protein:** 36.1 g
- **Fat:** 32.4 g
- **Sodium:** 165 mg

144. Lamb Roast

Preparation Time: 10 minutes
Cooking Time: 8 hours
Servings: 6
Ingredients:

- 2 ¼ lb. leg of lamb
- 3 carrots, sliced
- 1 onion, chopped
- 2 garlic cloves, minced
- 2 rosemary sprigs
- ½ cup red wine
- 1 beef stock cube
- Salt and pepper, to taste

Directions:

1. Season the lamb generously with salt and pepper.
2. Add the lamb to your Slow Cooker. Place the remaining ingredients in a bowl, crumble the stock cube inside, stir to combine, and pour over the lamb.
3. Add the rosemary sprigs inside and put the lid on.
4. Cook for 8 hours on LOW.
5. Open the lid and shred the lamb inside the pot. Stir to make sure it is equally moist.
6. Serve and enjoy!

Nutrition:

- **Calories:** 270 **Carbs:** 11 g
- **Protein:** 34 g
- **Total fats:** 7 g **Fiber:** 2 g

145. Pork Chops in Peach Glaze

Preparation Time: 10 minutes
Cooking Time: 16 minutes
Servings: 2
Ingredients:

- 2 (6-oz.) boneless pork chops, trimmed

- Sea salt and ground black pepper, as required
- ½ ripe yellow peach, peeled, pitted, and chopped
- 1 tbsp. olive oil
- 2 tbsp. shallot, minced
- 2 tbsp. garlic, minced
- 2 tbsp. fresh ginger, minced
- 4 to 6 drops of liquid stevia
- 1 tbsp. balsamic vinegar
- ¼ tsp. red pepper flakes, crushed
- ¼ cup filtered water

Directions:
1. Season the pork chops with sea salt and black pepper generously.
2. In a blender, add the peach pieces and pulse until puree forms.
3. Reserve the remaining peach pieces.
4. In a skillet, heat the oil over medium heat and sauté the shallots for about 1 to 2 minutes.
5. Add the garlic and ginger and sauté for about 1 minute.
6. Stir in the remaining ingredients and bring to a boil.
7. Now, reduce the heat to medium-low and simmer for about 4 to 5 minutes or until a sticky glaze forms.
8. Remove from the heat and reserve ⅓ of the glaze and set aside.
9. Coat the chops with the remaining glaze.
10. Heat a nonstick skillet over medium-high heat and sear the chops for about 4 minutes per side.
11. Transfer the chops onto a plate and coat with the remaining glaze evenly.
12. Serve immediately.

Meal prep tip: Transfer the pork chops into a large bowl and set them aside to cool. Divide the chops into 2 containers evenly. Cover the containers and refrigerate for 1 to 2 days. Reheat in the microwave before serving.

Nutrition:
- **Calories:** 359
- **Total carbs:** 12 g
- **Protein:** 46.2 g
- **Total fat:** 13.5 g
- **Saturated fat:** 3.2 g
- **Cholesterol:** 124 mg
- **Fiber:** 1.5 g
- **Sodium:** 102 mg
- **Potassium:** 938 mg

146. Spicy Chicken Drumsticks

Preparation Time: 15 minutes
Cooking Time: 3 hours
Servings: 4
Ingredients:
- Nonstick cooking spray
- 4 chicken drumsticks (about 1 lb. total), skinned*
- ½ cup bottled Picante sauce
- 2 tsp. bottled cayenne pepper sauce (such as Frank's Red Hot) or ⅛ tsp. cayenne pepper
- ½ tsp. smoked paprika
- ¼ tsp. dried thyme, crushed
- 1 bay leaf
- 2 tsp. olive oil

Directions:
1. Lightly coat an unheated 3- or 3 ½-quart slow cooker with cooking spray.
2. Place chicken in the bottom of the cooker. In a small bowl combine Picante sauce, pepper sauce, paprika, thyme, and bay leaf. Spoon over chicken in cooker.
3. Cover and cook on a low-heat setting for 6 hours or on a high-heat setting for 3 hours.
4. Transfer chicken pieces to a serving bowl. Remove bay leaf from sauce in cooker; stir in the oil.
5. Spoon sauce evenly over the chicken. Cover and let stand for 10 minutes to absorb flavors.
6. Spoon 1 tsp. sauce over each drumstick. Serve and enjoy

Nutrition:
- **Calories:** 241
- **Carbs:** 2.79 g
- **Protein:** 24.06 g
- **Fat:** 14.31 g

147. Beef and Chorizo Burger

Preparation Time: 25 minutes
Cooking Time: 0 minutes
Servings: 4
Ingredients:
- 5 slices pickled jalapeños; chopped
- ¼ lb. Mexican-style ground chorizo
- ¾ lb. 80/20 ground beef.
- ¼ cup chopped onion
- ¼ tsp. cumin
- 1 tsp. minced garlic
- 2 tsp. chili powder

Directions:
1. Take a large bowl, mix all ingredients. Divide the mixture into four sections and form them into burger patties.
2. Place burger patties into the air fryer basket, working in batches if necessary. Adjust the temperature to 375° F and set the timer for 15 minutes
3. Flip the patties halfway through the cooking time. Serve warm.

Nutrition:
- **Calories:** 291
- **Carbs:** 7 g
- **Protein:** 26 g
- **Fiber:** 9 g
- **Fat:** 13 g

148. Peppered Chicken Breast With Basil

Preparation Time: 10 minutes
Cooking Time: 20 minutes
Servings: 4
Ingredients:
- ¼ cup red bell peppers
- 1 cup chicken stock
- 2 pieces (no skin and bones) chicken breasts
- 4 pieces garlic cloves (crushed)
- 1 ½ tbsp. basil (crushed)

What you'll need from the store cupboard:
- 1 tbsp. chili powder

Directions:
1. In the instant pot, combine the ingredients and then

cover them and cook for 25 minutes at high temperature.
2. Release the pressure quickly for 5 minutes then split them among your plates before eating.

Nutrition:
- **Calories:** 230
- **Carbs:** 2.7 g
- **Protein:** 33.2 g
- **Fat:** 12.4 g
- **Fiber:** 0.8 g

149. Homemade Hamburgers

Preparation Time: 30 to 35 minutes
Cooking Time: 60 minutes
Servings: 6
Ingredients:
- ¼ cup barbecue sauce
- ¼ cup chopped onion
- ¼ cup ketchup
- ¼ tsp. pepper
- ½ cup fat-free milk
- ½ cup water
- 1 cup dry bread crumbs
- 1 lb. 90%-lean ground beef
- 1 tbsp. vinegar
- 1 tbsp. Worcestershire sauce
- 3 tbsp. maple sugar

Directions:
1. In a good-sized mixing vessel, moisten bread crumbs with milk.
2. Put in ground beef, onion, and pepper. Combine thoroughly. Set aside.
3. In a mixing vessel, make the sauce by mixing together completely maple sugar, vinegar, ketchup, Worcestershire sauce, barbecue sauce, and water.
4. Mold hamburger mixture into 6 patties.
5. Lay in a single layer in a baking dish.
6. Drizzle barbecue sauce over patties.
7. Cover and bake at 375° F for approximately half an hour.
8. Take out cover and bake another approximately half an hour, basting intermittently with sauce.

Nutrition:
- **Calories:** 255
- **Total carb:** 28 g
- **Protein:** 18 g
- **Total fat:** 7 g
- **Cholesterol:** 45 mg
- **Sodium:** 445 mg
- **Potassium:** 395 g
- **Dietary fiber:** 1 g
- **Phosphorus:** 190 g

150. Chicken Meatballs

Preparation Time: 5 minutes
Cooking Time: 26 minutes
Servings: 4
Ingredients:
- 1 lb. ground chicken
- 2 green onions, chopped
- ¾ tsp. ground black pepper
- ¼ cup shredded coconut, unsweetened
- 1 tsp. salt
- 1 tbsp. hoisin sauce
- 1 tbsp. soy sauce
- ½ cup cilantro, chopped
- 1 tsp. Sriracha sauce
- 1 tsp. sesame oil

Directions:
1. Switch on the air fryer, insert the fryer basket, grease it with olive oil, then shut with its lid, set the fryer at 350° F, and preheat for 5 minutes.
2. Meanwhile, place all the ingredients in a bowl, stir until well mixed and then shape the mixture into meatballs, 1 tsp. of chicken mixture per meatball.
3. Open the fryer, add chicken meatballs to it in a single layer, close with its lid and then spray with oil.
4. Cook the chicken meatballs for 10 minutes, flipping the meatballs halfway through, and then continue cooking for 3 minutes until golden.
5. When the air fryer beeps, open its lid, transfer chicken meatballs onto a serving plate and then cook the remaining meatballs in the same manner.
6. Serve straight away.

Nutrition:
- **Calories:** 223
- **Carbs:** 3 g
- **Protein:** 20 g
- **Fat:** 14 g
- **Fiber:** 1 g

CHAPTER 8:

Desserts

151. Flourless Chocolate Cake

Preparation Time: 10 minutes
Cooking Time: 45 minutes
Servings: 6
Ingredients:

- ½ cup of stevia
- 12 oz. unsweetened baking chocolate
- ⅔ cup of ghee
- ⅓ cup of warm water
- ¼ tsp. salt
- 4 large pastured eggs
- 2 cups of boiling water

Directions:

1. Line the bottom of a 9-inch pan of a springform with parchment paper.
2. Heat the water in a small pot; then add the salt and the stevia over the water until wait until the mixture becomes completely dissolved.
3. Melt the baking chocolate into a double boiler or simply microwave it for about 30 seconds.
4. Mix the melted chocolate and the butter in a large bowl with an electric mixer.
5. Beat in your hot mixture; then crack in the egg and whisk after adding each of the eggs.
6. Pour the obtained mixture into your prepared springform tray.
7. Wrap the springform tray with foil paper.
8. Place the springform tray in a large cake tray and add boiling water right to the outside; make sure the depth doesn't exceed 1 inch.
9. Bake the cake into the water bath for about 45 minutes at a temperature of about 350° F.
10. Remove the tray from the boiling water and transfer it to a wire to cool.
11. Let the cake chill overnight in the refrigerator.

Nutrition:

- **Calories:** 295
- **Carbs:** 6 g
- **Fiber:** 4 g

152. Peanut Butter Cups

Preparation Time: 5 minutes
Cooking Time: 10 minutes
Servings: 4
Ingredients:

- 1 packet plain gelatin
- ¼ cup honey

- 2 cups nonfat cream
- ½ tsp. vanilla
- ¼ cup low-fat peanut butter
- 2 tbsp. unsalted peanuts, chopped

Directions:
1. Mix gelatin, honey, and cream in a pan.
2. Let sit for 5 minutes.
3. Place over medium heat and cook until gelatin has been dissolved.
4. Stir in vanilla and peanut butter.
5. Pour into custard cups. Chill for 3 hours.
6. Top with the peanuts and serve.

Nutrition:
- **Calories:** 171 **Carbs:** 21 g
- **Protein:** 6.8 g

153. Ice Cream Brownie Cake

Preparation Time: 5 minutes
Cooking Time: 10 minutes
Servings: 4
Ingredients:
- Cooking spray
- 12 oz. no-sugar brownie mix - ¼ cup oil
- 2 egg whites - 3 tbsp. water
- 2 cups sugar-free ice cream

Directions:
1. Preheat your oven to 325° F.
2. Spray your baking pan with oil.
3. Mix brownie mix, oil, egg whites, and water in a bowl.
4. Pour into the baking pan.
5. Bake for 25 minutes. Let cool. Freeze brownie for 2 hours. Spread ice cream over the brownie. Freeze for 8 hours.

Nutrition:
- **Calories:** 198
- **Carbs:** 33g
- **Protein:** 3 g

154. Fruit Pizza

Preparation Time: 5 minutes
Cooking Time: 10 minutes
Servings: 4
Ingredients:
- 1 tsp. maple syrup
- ¼ tsp. vanilla extract
- ½ cup coconut milk yogurt
- 2 round slices of watermelon
- ½ cup blackberries, sliced
- ½ cup strawberries, sliced
- 2 tbsp. coconut flakes (unsweetened)

Directions:
1. Mix maple syrup, vanilla, and yogurt in a bowl.
2. Spread the mixture on top of the watermelon slice.
3. Top with the berries and coconut flakes.

Nutrition:
- **Calories:** 70
- **Carbs:** 14.6 g
- **Protein:** 1.2 g

155. Choco Peppermint Cake

Preparation Time: 5 minutes
Cooking Time: 10 minutes
Servings: 4
Ingredients:
- Cooking spray
- ⅓ cup oil

- 15 oz. package chocolate cake mix
- 3 eggs, beaten
- 1 cup water
- ¼ tsp. peppermint extract

Directions:
1. Spray slow cooker with oil.
2. Mix all the ingredients in a bowl.
3. Use an electric mixer on a medium-speed setting to mix ingredients for 2 minutes.
4. Pour the mixture into the slow cooker.
5. Cover the pot and cook on low for 3 hours.
6. Let cool before slicing and serving.

Nutrition:
- **Calories:** 185
- **Carbs:** 27g
- **Protein:** 3.8g

156. Roasted Mango

Preparation Time: 5 minutes
Cooking Time: 10 minutes
Servings: 4
Ingredients:

- 2 mangoes, sliced
- 2 tsp. crystallized ginger, chopped
- 2 tsp. orange zest
- 2 tbsp. coconut flakes (unsweetened)

Directions:
1. Preheat your oven to 350° F.
2. Add mango slices in custard cups.
3. Top with ginger, orange zest, and coconut flakes.
4. Bake in the oven for 10 minutes.

Nutrition:
- **Calories:** 89
- **Carbs:** 20 g
- **Protein:** 0.8 g

157. Figs With Honey & Yogurt

Preparation Time: 5 minutes
Cooking Time: 10 minutes
Servings: 4
Ingredients:

- ½ tsp. vanilla
- 8 oz. nonfat yogurt
- 2 figs, sliced
- 1 tbsp. walnuts, chopped and toasted
- 2 tsp. honey

Directions:
1. Stir vanilla into yogurt.
2. Mix well.
3. Top with the figs and sprinkle with walnuts.
4. Drizzle with honey and serve.

Nutrition:
- **Calories:** 157
- **Carbs:** 24 g
- **Protein:** 7 g

158. Raspberry Cake With White Chocolate Sauce

Preparation Time: 15 minutes
Cooking Time: 60 minutes
Servings: 5
Ingredients:

- 5 oz. melted cacao butter
- 2 oz. grass-fed ghee
- ½ cup coconut cream
- 1 cup green banana flour
- 3 tsp. pure vanilla

- 4 large eggs
- ½ cup as lakanto monk fruit
- 1 tsp. baking powder
- 2 tsp. apple cider vinegar
- 2 cups raspberries

White chocolate sauce:

- 3 ½ oz. cacao butter
- ½ cup coconut cream
- 2 tsp. pure vanilla extract
- 1 pinch of salt

Directions:

1. Preheat your oven to a temperature of about 280° F.
2. Combine the green banana flour with the pure vanilla extract, baking powder, coconut cream, eggs, cider vinegar, and the monk fruit and mix very well.
3. Leave the raspberries aside and line a cake loaf tin with baking paper.
4. Pour the batter into the baking tray and scatter the raspberries over the top of the cake.
5. Place the tray in your oven and bake it for about 60 minutes.

Make the sauce:

1. Combine the cacao cream, vanilla extract, cacao butter, and salt in a saucepan over low heat.
2. Mix all your ingredients with a fork to make sure the cacao butter mixes very well with the cream.
3. Remove from the heat and set aside to cool a little bit, but don't let it harden.
4. Drizzle with the chocolate sauce.
5. Scatter the cake with more raspberries.

6. Slice your cake; then serve and enjoy it!

Nutrition:

- **Calories:** 323
- **Carbs:** 9.9 g
- **Fiber:** 4 g

159. Berry Almond Parfait

Preparation Time: 10 minutes
Cooking Time: 30 minutes
Servings: 4
Ingredients:

- 1 to 8 oz. container plain yogurt, low-fat and drained
- 1 cup of sliced strawberries
- ½ cup raspberries
- ½ cup blueberries
- ⅛ tsp. almond extract
- 1 tbsp. honey + 2 tsp., divided
- 2 tbsp. toasted slivered almonds for toppings

Directions:

1. Drain and thicken yogurt in the fridge using a paper towel-lined strainer for 2 to 24 hours. (Do this the night before).
2. Combine all ingredients but using only 2 tsp. of honey. Toss lightly to mix. Chill for 30 minutes to 2 hours.
3. Transfer the drained yogurt to a bowl and stir in the remaining honey.
4. Layer ⅓ cup of berries mixture and half yogurt alternately in 2 parfait glasses.
5. Top with almonds to serve.

Nutrition:
- **Calories:** 220
- **Carbs:** 30 g
- **Protein:** 9 g
- **Fats:** 6 g
- **Fiber:** 6 g
- **Sodium:** 84 mg

160. Cappuccino Cupcakes

Preparation Time: 10 minutes
Cooking Time: 30 minutes
Servings: 17
Ingredients:
- 2 eggs
- 2 cups all-purpose flour
- ¼ cup instant coffee granules
- ½ cup of baby food
- ½ cup cocoa, crushed

What you will need from the store cupboard:
- ¼ cup canola oil
- 1 tsp. baking soda
- 2 tsp. vanilla extract
- ½ tsp. salt
- 1 ½ cups low-fat whipped topping
- ½ cup hot water

Directions:
1. Bring together the cocoa, flour, salt, and baking soda in your bowl.
2. Dissolve the coffee granules in hot water.
3. Now whisk together the baby food, eggs, coffee mix, and vanilla in a bowl.
4. Stir the dry ingredients in gradually.
5. Fill into your muffin cups.
6. Bake for 10 to 12 minutes.
7. Sprinkle with cocoa and add the whipped toppings before serving.

Nutrition:
- **Calories:** 192
- **Carbs:** 33 g
- **Protein:** 3 g
- **Total fat:** 5 g
- **Fiber:** 1 g
- **Cholesterol:** 22 mg

161. Pumpkin Spiced Almonds

Preparation Time: 10 minutes
Cooking Time: 30 minutes
Servings: 4
Ingredients:
- 1 tbsp. olive oil
- 1 ¼ tsp. pumpkin pie spice
- Pinch salt
- 1 cup whole almonds, raw

Directions:
1. Preheat the oven to 300° F and line a baking sheet with parchment.
2. Whisk together the olive oil, pumpkin pie spice, and salt in a mixing bowl.
3. Toss in the almonds until evenly coated, then spread on the baking sheet.
4. Bake for 25 minutes then cool completely and store in an airtight container.

Nutrition:
- **Calories:** 170
- **Carbs:** 5.5 g
- **Protein:** 5 g
- **Fat:** 15.5 g
- **Fiber:** 3 g
- **Net carbs:** 2.5 g

162. Pumpkin Custard

Preparation Time: 10 minutes
Cooking Time: 30 minutes
Servings: 6
Ingredients:
- ½ cup almond flour
- 4 eggs
- 1 cup pumpkin puree
- ½ cup stevia
- ⅛ tsp. sea salt
- 1 tsp. vanilla extract or maple flavoring
- 4 tbsp. butter, ghee, or coconut oil melted
- 1 tsp. pumpkin pie spice
- ¼ cup nutmeg
- Whipped cream as desired

Directions:
1. Grease or spray a slow cooker with butter or coconut oil spray.
2. In a medium mixing bowl, beat the eggs until smooth. Then add in the sweetener.
3. To the egg mixture, add in the pumpkin puree along with vanilla or maple extract.
4. Then add almond flour to the mixture along with the pumpkin pie spice and salt. Add melted butter, coconut oil, or ghee.
5. Transfer the mixture into a slow cooker. Close the lid. Cook for 2 to 2 ¾ hours on low.
6. When through, serve with whipped cream, and then sprinkle with little nutmeg if need be.
7. Set slow-cooker to the low setting. Cook for 2 to 2.45 hours, and begin checking at the two-hour mark. Serve warm with stevia-sweetened whipped cream and a sprinkle of nutmeg.

Nutrition:
- **Calories:** 147
- **Total carbs:** 4 g
- **Protein:** 5 g
- **Fat:** 12 g

163. Strawberry Shake

Preparation Time: 10 minutes
Cooking Time: 30 minutes
Servings: 2
Ingredients:
- 1 ½ cups fresh strawberries, hulled
- 1 large frozen banana, peeled
- 2 scoops of unsweetened vegan vanilla protein powder
- 2 tbsp. hemp seeds
- 2 cups unsweetened hemp milk

Directions:
1. In a high-speed blender, place all the ingredients and pulse until creamy.
2. Pour into two glasses and serve immediately.

Nutrition:
- **Calories:** 325
- **Total carbs:** 23.3 g
- **Protein:** 31.2 g
- **Total fat:** 13 g
- **Saturated fat:** 0.8 g
- **Cholesterol:** 0 mg
- **Sodium:** 391 mg
- **Fiber:** 3.9 g

164. Cinnamon Protein Bars

Preparation Time: 10 minutes
Cooking Time: 30 minutes
Servings: 8
Ingredients:

- 2 scoops of vanilla protein powder
- ¼ cup coconut oil, melted
- 1 cup almond butter
- ¼ tsp. cinnamon
- 12 drops liquid stevia
- Pinch of salt

Directions:

1. In a bowl, mix together all ingredients until well combined.
2. Transfer bar mixture into a baking dish and press down evenly.
3. Place in refrigerator until firm.
4. Slice and serve.

Nutrition:

- **Calories:** 99
- **Carbs:** 0.6 g
- **Protein:** 7.2 g
- **Fat:** 8 g
- **Cholesterol:** 0 mg

165. Chocó Cookies

Preparation Time: 10 minutes
Cooking Time: 30 minutes
Servings: 14
Ingredients:

- 1 egg
- ½ cup stevia
- ¼ cup unsweetened cocoa powder
- 1 cup almond butter
- 3 tbsp. unsweetened almond milk
- ¼ cup unsweetened chocolate chips

Directions:

1. Preheat the oven to 350° F/ 180° C.
2. Line baking tray with parchment paper and set aside.
3. In a bowl, mix together almond butter, egg, sweetener, almond milk, and cocoa powder until well combined.
4. Stir in Chocó chips.
5. Make cookies from the mixture and place them on a baking tray.
6. Bake for 10 minutes.
7. Allow to cool completely, then serve.

Nutrition:

- **Calories:** 44
- **Carbs:** 2.2 g
- **Protein:** 1.5 g
- **Fat:** 3.5 g
- **Cholesterol:** 12 mg

166. Chocolate Avocado Ice Cream

Preparation Time: 10 minutes
Cooking Time: 30 minutes
Servings: 6
Ingredients:

- 2 large organic avocados, pitted
- ½ cup coconut sugar
- ½ cup cocoa powder, organic and unsweetened
- 25 drops of liquid stevia
- 2 tsp. vanilla extract, unsweetened
- 1 cup coconut milk, full-fat and unsweetened

- ½ cup heavy whipping cream, full-fat
- 6 squares of chocolate, unsweetened and chopped

Directions:
1. Scoop out the flesh from each avocado, place it in a bowl and add vanilla, milk, and cream and blend using an immersion blender until smooth and creamy.
2. Add remaining ingredients except for chocolate and mix until well combined and smooth.
3. Fold in chopped chocolate and let the mixture chill in the refrigerator for 8 to 12 hours or until cooled.
4. When ready to serve, let ice cream stand for 30 minutes at room temperature, then process it using an ice cream machine as per manufacturer instruction.
5. Serve immediately.

Nutrition:
- **Calories:** 216.7
- **Net carbs:** 3.7 g
- **Protein:** 3.8 g
- **Fat:** 19.4 g
- **Fiber:** 7.4 g

167. Cheese Crisp Crackers

Preparation Time: 10 minutes
Cooking Time: 30 minutes
Servings: 4
Ingredients:
- 4 slices pepper jack cheese, quartered
- 4 slices Colby jack cheese, quartered
- 4 slices cheddar cheese, quartered

Directions:
1. Heat oven to 400° F. Line a cooking sheet with parchment paper.
2. Place cheese in a single layer on a prepared pan and bake for 10 minutes, or until cheese gets firm.
3. Transfer to paper towel line surface to absorb excess oil. Let cool, cheese will crisp up more as it cools.
4. Store in an airtight container, or Ziploc bag. Serve with your favorite dip or salsa.

Nutrition:
- **Calories:** 253
- **Total carbs:** 1 g
- **Protein:** 15 g
- **Fat:** 20 g
- **Fiber:** 0 g

168. Coconut Milk Shakes

Preparation Time: 10 minutes
Cooking Time: 30 minutes
Servings: 2
Ingredients:
- 1 ½ cup vanilla ice cream
- ½ cup coconut milk, unsweetened

What you'll need from the store cupboard:
- 2 ½ tbsp. coconut flakes
- 1 tsp. unsweetened cocoa

Directions:
1. Heat oven to 350° F.
2. Place coconut on a baking sheet and bake, 2 to 3 minutes, stirring often, until coconut is toasted.

3. Place ice cream, milk, 2 tbsp. of coconut, and cocoa in a blender and process until smooth.
4. Pour into glasses and garnish with remaining toasted coconut. Serve immediately.

Nutrition:
- **Calories:** 323
- **Total carbs:** 23 g
- **Net carbs:** 19 g
- **Protein:** 3 g **Fat:** 24 g
- **Fiber:** 4 g

169. Lava Cake

Preparation Time: 10 minutes
Cooking Time: 10 minutes
Servings: 2
Ingredients:

- 2 oz. dark chocolate; you should at least use chocolate of 85% cocoa solids
- 1 tbsp. super-fine almond flour
- 2 oz. unsalted almond butter
- 2 large eggs

Directions:
1. Heat your oven to a temperature of about 350° F.
2. Grease 2 heat-proof ramekins with almond butter.
3. Now, melt the chocolate and the almond butter and stir very well.
4. Beat the eggs very well with a mixer.
5. Add the eggs to the chocolate and the butter mixture and mix very well with almond flour and the swerve; then stir.
6. Pour the dough into 2 ramekins.
7. Bake for about 9 to 10 minutes.
8. Turn the cakes over plates and serve with pomegranate seeds!

Nutrition:
- **Calories:** 459 **Carbs:** 3.5 g
- **Fiber:** 0.8 g

170. Cheese Cake

Preparation Time: 15 minutes
Cooking Time: 50 minutes
Servings: 6
Ingredients:
Almond flour cheesecake crust:

- 2 cups blanched almond flour
- ⅓ cup almond butter
- 3 tbsp. maple syrup
- 1 tsp. vanilla extract

Keto cheesecake filling:

- 32 oz. softened cream cheese
- 1 ¼ cups maple syrup
- 3 large eggs
- 1 tbsp. lemon juice
- 1 tsp. vanilla extract

Directions:
1. Preheat your oven to a temperature of about 350° F.
2. Grease a springform pan of 9" with cooking spray or just line its bottom with parchment paper.
3. In order to make the cheesecake crust, stir in the melted butter, the almond flour, the vanilla extract, and the maple syrup in a large bowl.
4. The dough will get will be a bit crumbly; so, press it into

the bottom of your prepared tray.
5. Bake for about 12 minutes; then let cool for about 10 minutes.
6. In the meantime, beat the softened cream cheese and the powdered sweetener at a low speed until it becomes smooth.
7. Crack in the eggs and beat them in at a low to medium speed until it becomes fluffy. Make sure to add one at a time.
8. Add in the lemon juice and the vanilla extract and mix at a low to medium speed with a mixer.
9. Pour your filling into your pan right on top of the crust. You can use a spatula to smooth the top of the cake.
10. Bake for about 45 to 50 minutes.
11. Remove the baked cheesecake from your oven and run a knife around its edge.
12. Let the cake cool for about 4 hours in the refrigerator.
13. Serve and enjoy your delicious cheesecake!

Nutrition:
- **Calories:** 325 **Carbs:** 6 g
- **Fiber:** 1 g

171. Cake With Whipped Cream Icing

Preparation Time: 20 minutes
Cooking Time: 25 minutes
Servings: 7
Ingredients:
- ¾ cup coconut flour
- ¾ cup swerve sweetener
- ½ cup cocoa powder
- 2 tsp. baking powder
- 6 large eggs
- ⅔ cup heavy whipping cream
- ½ cup melted almond butter

Whipped cream icing:
- 1 cup heavy whipping cream
- ¼ cup swerve sweetener
- 1 tsp. vanilla extract
- ⅓ cup sifted cocoa powder

Directions:
1. Preheat your oven to a temperature of about 350° F.
2. Grease an 8x8 cake tray with cooking spray.
3. Add the coconut flour, swerve sweetener; cocoa powder, baking powder, eggs, melted butter; and combine very well with an electric or a hand mixer.
4. Pour your batter into the cake tray and bake for about 25 minutes.
5. Remove the cake tray from the oven and let cool for about 5 minutes.

Make the icing:
1. Whip the cream until it becomes fluffy; then add in the swerve, the vanilla, and the cocoa powder.
2. Add the swerve, the vanilla, and the cocoa powder; then continue mixing until your ingredients are very well combined. Frost your baked cake with the icing!

Nutrition:
- **Calories:** 357 **Carbs:** 11 g
- **Fiber:** 2 g

172. Walnut-Fruit Cake

Preparation Time: 15 minutes
Cooking Time: 20 minutes
Servings: 7
Ingredients:

- ½ cup almond butter (softened)
- ¼ cup maple sugar
- ¼ cup coconut oil
- 1 tbsp. ground cinnamon
- ½ tsp. ground nutmeg
- ¼ tsp. ground cloves
- 4 large pastured eggs
- 1 tsp. vanilla extract
- ½ tsp. almond extract
- 2 cups almond flour
- ½ cup chopped walnuts
- ¼ cup dried of unsweetened cranberries
- ¼ cup seedless raisins

Directions:

1. Preheat your oven to a temperature of about 350° F and grease an 8-inch baking tin of round shape with coconut oil.
2. Beat the maple sugar at a high speed until it becomes fluffy.
3. Add the cinnamon, nutmeg, and cloves; then blend your ingredients until they become smooth.
4. Crack in the eggs and beat very well by adding one at a time, plus the almond extract and the vanilla.
5. Whisk in the almond flour until it forms a smooth batter then fold in the nuts and the fruit.
6. Spread your mixture into your prepared baking pan and bake it for about 20 minutes.
7. Remove the cake from the oven and let cool for about 5 minutes.
8. Dust the cake with powdered maple sugar.

Nutrition:

- **Calories:** 250 **Carbs:** 12 g
- **Fiber:** 2 g

173. Dark Chocolate Cake

Preparation Time: 10 minutes
Cooking Time: 30 minutes
Servings: 10
Ingredients:

- 1 cup almond flour
- 3 eggs
- 2 tbsp. almond flour
- ¼ tsp. salt
- ½ cup swerve granular
- ¾ tsp. vanilla extract
- ⅔ cup almond milk, unsweetened
- ½ cup cocoa powder
- 6 tbsp. butter, melted
- 1 ½ tsp. baking powder
- 3 tbsp. unflavored whey protein powder or egg white protein powder
- ⅓ cup sugar-free chocolate chips, optional

Directions:

1. Grease the slow cooker well.
2. Whisk the almond flour together with cocoa powder, sweetener, whey protein powder, salt, and baking powder in a bowl. Then stir in butter along with almond milk, eggs, and the vanilla extract until well combined,

and then stir in the chocolate chips if desired.
3. When done, pour into the slow cooker. Allow cooking for 2 to 2 ½ hours on low.
4. When through, turn off the slow cooker and let the cake cool for about 20 to 30 minutes.
5. When cooled, cut the cake into pieces and serve warm with lightly sweetened whipped cream. Enjoy!

Nutrition:
- **Calories:** 205
- **Total carbs:** 8.4 g
- **Protein:** 12 g **Fat:** 17 g

174. Strawberry & Watermelon Pops

Preparation Time: 10 minutes
Cooking Time: 30 minutes
Servings: 6
Ingredients:
- ¾ cup strawberries, sliced
- 2 cups watermelon, cubed
- ¼ cup lime juice
- 2 tbsp. coconut sugar
- ⅛ tsp. salt

Directions:
1. Put the strawberries inside popsicle molds.
2. In a blender, pulse the rest of the ingredients until well mixed. Pour the puree into a sieve before pouring it into the molds.
3. Freeze for 6 hours.

Nutrition:
- **Calories:** 57 **Protein:** 1 g
- **Total carbs:** 14 g

- **Total fat:** 0 g
- **Saturated fat:** 0 g
- **Cholesterol:** 0 mg
- **Sodium:** 180 mg
- **Dietary fiber:** 2 g
- **Potassium:** 180 mg

175. Baked Apples With Dried Fruit

Preparation Time: 10 minutes
Cooking Time: 1 hour
Servings: 4
Ingredients:
- 4 large apple s, cored to make a cavity
- 4 tsp. raisins or cranberries
- 4 tsp. pure maple syrup
- ½ tsp. ground cinnamon
- ½ cup unsweetened apple juice or water

Directions:
1. Preheat the oven to 350° F.
2. Place apples in a baking pan that will hold them upright. Put the dried fruit into the cavities and drizzle with maple syrup. Sprinkle with cinnamon. Pour apple juice or water on the apples.
3. Cover loosely with foil and bake for 50 minutes to 1 hour, or until the apples are tender when pierced with a fork.

Serving suggestion: Serve the apples topped with vegan whipped cream.

Nutrition:
- **Calories:** 158
- **Carbs:** 42 g
- **Fat:** 1 g
- **Protein:** 1 g

176. Raspberry Almond Tart

Preparation Time: 10 minutes
Cooking Time: 30 minutes
Servings: 4
Ingredients:

- 5 egg whites
- 1 tsp. vanilla
- 1 ½ cups raspberries
- 1 lemon zest, grated
- 1 cup almond flour
- ½ cup swerve
- ½ cup butter, melted
- 1 tsp. baking powder

Directions:

1. Preheat the oven to 375° F/ 190° C.
2. Grease tart tin with cooking spray and set aside.
3. In a large bowl, whisk egg whites until foamy.
4. Add sweetener, baking powder, vanilla, lemon zest, and almond flour and mix until well combined.
5. Add melted butter and stir well.
6. Pour batter in tart tin and top with raspberries.
7. Bake in preheated oven for 20 to 23 minutes.
8. Serve and enjoy.

Nutrition:

- **Calories:** 378
- **Carbs:** 14 g
- **Protein:** 11 g
- **Fat:** 8 g
- **Cholesterol:** 0 mg

177. Oatmeal Butterscotch Cookies

Preparation Time: 10 minutes
Cooking Time: 30 minutes
Servings: 4
Ingredients:

- ½ tsp. cinnamon, ground
- 3 cups oats
- 2 eggs

What you will need from the store cupboard:

- 1 tsp. baking soda
- 1-¼ all-purpose flour
- 1 cup margarine or butter
- 1 tsp. vanilla extract
- ½ tsp. salt

Directions:

1. Preheat your oven to 350° F.
2. Bring together the baking soda, flour, salt, and cinnamon in a bowl.
3. Beat the eggs, vanilla extract, and butter in a mixer bowl.
4. Beat in the flour mix gradually.
5. Stir in the oats.
6. Place rounded tbsp. on baking sheets. Bake for 5 to 6 minutes.
7. Let it cool for a couple of minutes.

Nutrition:

- **Calories:** 130
- **Carbs:** 16 g
- **Protein:** 1 g
- **Fat:** 7 g
- **Cholesterol:** 20 mg
- **Sodium:** 90 mg

178. Avocado Mousse

Preparation Time: 10 minutes
Cooking Time: 30 minutes
Servings: 3
Ingredients:

- 2 ripe Haas avocados, peeled, pitted, and chopped roughly
- 1 tsp. liquid stevia
- 1 tsp. organic vanilla extract
- Pinch of salt

Directions:
1. In a high-speed blender, add all the ingredients and pulse until smooth.
2. Transfer the pudding into a serving bowl.
3. Cover the bowl and refrigerate to chill for at least 2 hours before serving.

Meal prep tip: Transfer the mousse into an airtight container. Cover the containers and refrigerate for about 1 day.

Nutrition:
- Calories: 277
- Total carbs: 11.7 g
- Protein: 2.6 g
- Total fat: 26.1 g
- Saturated fat: 5.5 g
- Cholesterol: 0 mg
- Fiber: 8 g **Sodium:** 59 mg
- Potassium: 652 mg

179. Cinnamon Toasted Almonds

Preparation Time: 10 minutes
Cooking Time: 30 minutes
Servings: 8
Ingredients:

- 2 cups whole almonds
- 1 tbsp. olive oil
- 1 tsp. ground cinnamon
- ½ tsp. salt

Directions:
1. Preheat the oven to 325° F and line a baking sheet with parchment.
2. Toss together the almonds, olive oil, cinnamon, and salt.
3. Spread the almonds on the baking sheet in a single layer.
4. Bake for 25 minutes, stirring several times until toasted.

Nutrition:
- Calories: 150
- Total carbs: 5.3 g
- Net carbs: 2.2 g
- Protein: 5 g
- Total fat: 13.6 g
- Saturated fat: 1.2 g
- Fiber: 3.1 g
- Sodium: 148 mg

180. Cinnamon Apple Chips

Preparation Time: 10 minutes
Cooking Time: 30 minutes
Servings: 2
Ingredients:

- 1 medium apple, sliced thin

What you'll need from the store cupboard:

- ¼ tsp. cinnamon
- ¼ tsp. nutmeg
- Nonstick cooking spray

Directions:
1. Heat oven to 375° F. Spray a baking sheet with cooking spray.
2. Place apples in a mixing bowl and add spices. Toss to coat.
3. Arrange apples, in a single layer, on the prepared pan.

Bake 4 minutes, turn apples over, and bake 4 minutes more.
4. Serve immediately or store in an airtight container.

Nutrition:
- Calories: 58
- Total carbs: 15 g
- Protein: 0 g Fat: 0 g
- Fiber: 3 g

181. Dark Chocolate Almond Yogurt Cups

Preparation Time: 10 minutes
Cooking Time: 0 minutes
Servings: 6
Ingredients:
- 3 cups plain nonfat Greek yogurt
- ½ tsp. almond extract
- ¼ tsp. liquid stevia extract (more to taste)
- 2 oz. 70% dark chocolate, chopped
- ½ cup slivered almonds

Directions:
1. Whisk together the yogurt, almond extract, and liquid stevia in a medium bowl.
2. Spoon the yogurt into four dessert cups.
3. Sprinkle with chopped chocolate and slivered almonds.

Nutrition:
- Calories: 170
- Total carbs: 14.7 g
- Net carbs: 12.2 g
- Protein: 2.1 g
- Total fat: 0.7 g
- Saturated fat: 0.1 g
- Fiber: 2.5 g
- Sodium: 41 mg

182. Tomato & Cheese in Lettuce Packets

Preparation Time: 10 minutes
Cooking Time: 30 minutes
Servings: 36
Ingredients:
- ¼ lb. Gruyere cheese, grated
- ¼ lb. feta cheese, crumbled
- ½ tsp. oregano
- 1 tomato, chopped
- ½ cup buttermilk
- ½ head lettuce

Directions:
1. In a bowl, mix feta and Gruyere cheese, oregano, tomato, and buttermilk.
2. Separate the lettuce leaves and put them on a serving platter. Divide the mixture between them, roll up, folding in the ends to secure and serve.

Nutrition:
- Calories: 433
- Net carbs: 6.6 g
- Protein: 27.5 g
- Fat: 32.5 g

183. Mango Mousse

Preparation Time: 10 minutes
Cooking Time: 30 minutes
Servings: 6
Ingredients:
- 1 banana
- 2 mangoes, seeded, cubed, and peeled
- ⅔ cup plain yogurt
- 1 cup low-fat milk
- ⅛ cup unsweetened coconut

What you will need from the store cupboard:

- 1 tsp. vanilla extract
- 6 ice cubes
- 2 tsp. honey

Directions:
1. Bring together the vanilla extract, yogurt, honey, low-fat milk, unsweetened coconut, ice cubes, mangoes, and banana in your blender.
2. Blend until it becomes smooth.
3. Refrigerate for a couple of hours.
4. Pour into each dish before serving.

Nutrition:
- **Calories:** 87
- **Carbs:** 20 g
- **Protein:** 2 g
- **Total fat:** 0 g
- **Fiber:** 2 g
- **Cholesterol:** 1 mg

184. Banana Split Sundae

Preparation Time: 10 minutes
Cooking Time: 30 minutes
Servings: 4
Ingredients:

- 3 frozen, sliced overripe bananas (see Tip)
- 2 tbsp. peanut butter
- 1 tbsp. thawed frozen light whipped topping
- 1 tsp. sugar-free chocolate-flavor syrup
- 1 tsp. chopped peanuts
- 1 maraschino cherry

Directions:
1. Combine peanut butter and bananas in a food processor. Process with cover until almost no lumps remain. Scoop the mixture into sundae dishes.
2. Garnish top with whipped topping, maraschino cherry, peanuts, and sugar-free chocolate-flavor syrup. Serve right away.

Nutrition:
- **Calories:** 166
- **Total carbs:** 27 g
- **Protein:** 3 g
- **Total fat:** 6 g
- **Saturated fat:** 2 g
- **Cholesterol:** 0 mg
- **Fiber:** 3 g
- **Sodium:** 60 mg

185. Tzatziki Dip With Cauliflower

Preparation Time: 10 minutes
Cooking Time: 0 minutes
Servings: 6
Ingredients:

- ½ (8-oz.) package cream cheese, softened
- 1 cup sour cream
- 1 tbsp. ranch seasoning
- 1 English cucumber, diced
- 2 tbsp. chopped chives
- 2 cups cauliflower florets

Directions:
1. Beat the cream cheese with an electric mixer until creamy.
2. Add the sour cream and ranch seasoning, then beat until smooth.

3. Fold in the cucumbers and chives, then chill before serving with cauliflower florets for dipping.

Nutrition:
- **Calories:** 125
- **Carbs:** 5.5 g
- **Net carbs:** 4.5 g
- **Protein:** 3 g
- **Fat:** 10.5 g
- **Fiber:** 1 g

186. Rustic Pear Pie With Nuts

Preparation Time: 10 minutes
Cooking Time: 40 minutes
Servings: 4
Ingredients:
Cake:

- 100 g all-purpose flour
- 1 g of salt
- 12 g maple sugar
- 84 g unsalted butter, cold, cut into 13 mm pieces
- 30 ml of water, frozen
- 1 egg, beaten
- 12 g turbinated sugar
- Nonstick spray oil
- 20 g of honey
- 5 ml of water
- Roasted nuts, chopped, to decorate, as desired

Filling:

- 1 large pear, peeled, finely sliced
- 5 g cornstarch
- 24 g maple sugar
- 1 g ground cinnamon
- A pinch salt

Directions:
1. Mix 90 g of flour, salt, and maple sugar in a large bowl until well combined. Join the butter in the mixture using a pastry mixer or food processor until thick crumbs form. Add cold water and mix until it joins. Shape the dough into a bowl, cover with plastic and let cool in the refrigerator for 1 hour.
2. Mix the stuffing ingredients in a bowl until they are combined. Roll a roll through your cooled dough until it is 216 mm in diameter. Add 10 g of flour on top of the dough leaving 38 mm without flour. Place the pear slices in decorative circles superimposed on the floured part of the crust. Remove any remaining pear juice on the slices. Fold the edge over the filling.
3. Cover the edges with beaten eggs and sprinkle the maple sugar over the whole cake. Set aside
4. Preheat the air fryer set the temperature to 160° C. Spray the preheated air fryer with oil spray and place the cake inside. Set the time to 45 minutes at 160° C. Mix the honey and water and pass the mixture through the cake when you finish cooking.
5. Garnish with toasted chopped nuts.

Nutrition:
- **Calories:** 20
- **Carbs:** 0 g
- **Protein:** 0 g
- **Fat:** 0 g
- **Cholesterol:** 0 mg

187. Raspberry Peach Cobbler

Preparation Time: 10 minutes
Cooking Time: 40 minutes
Servings: 8
Ingredients:

- 1 ¼ lbs. peaches, peeled and sliced
- 2 cups fresh raspberries
- ½ cup low-fat buttermilk
- 2 tbsp. cold margarine, cut into pieces
- 1 tsp lemon zest

What you'll need from the store cupboard:

- ¾ cup + 2 tbsp. flour, divided
- 4 tbsp. + 2 tsp maple sugar, divided
- ½ tsp. baking powder
- ½ tsp. baking soda
- ⅛ tsp. salt
- Nonstick cooking spray

Directions:

1. Heat oven to 425° F. Spray an 11×7-inch baking dish with cooking spray.
2. In a large bowl, stir together 2 tbsp. of maple sugar and 2 tbsp. of flour. Add the fruit and zest and toss to coat. Pour into prepared baking dish. Bake 15 minutes, or until fruit is bubbling around the edges.
3. In a medium bowl, combine remaining flour, 2 tbsp. of maple sugar, baking powder, baking soda, and salt. Cut in margarine with a pastry cutter until it resembles coarse crumbs. Stir in the buttermilk just until moistened.
4. Remove the fruit from the oven and top with dollops of the buttermilk mixture. Sprinkle the remaining 2 tsp. of maple sugar over the top and bake 18 to 20 minutes or top is lightly browned. Serve warm.

Nutrition:

- **Calories:** 130
- **Total carbs:** 22 g
- **Net carbs:** 19 g
- **Protein:** 2 g
- **Fat:** 3 g
- **Fiber:** 3 g

188. Apricot Soufflé

Preparation Time: 10 minutes
Cooking Time: 40 minutes
Servings: 6
Ingredients:

- 4 egg whites
- 3 egg yolks, beaten
- 3 tbsp. margarine

What you'll need from the store cupboard:

- ¾ cup sugar-free apricot fruit spread
- ⅓ cup dried apricots, diced fine
- ¼ cup warm water
- 2 tbsp. flour
- ¼ tsp. cream of tartar
- ⅛ tsp. salt

Directions:

1. Heat oven to 325° F.
2. In a medium saucepan, over medium heat, melt margarine. Stir in flour and cook, stirring, until bubbly.

3. Stir together the fruit spread and water in a small bowl and add it to the saucepan with the apricots. Cook, stirring, 3 minutes or until mixture thickens.
4. Remove from heat and whisk in egg yolks. Let cool to room temperature, stirring occasionally.
5. In a medium bowl, beat egg whites, salt, and cream of tartar at high speed until stiff peaks form. Gently fold into cooled apricot mixture.
6. Spoon into a 1 ½ quart soufflé dish. Bake 30 minutes, or until puffed and golden brown. Serve immediately.

Nutrition:
- **Calories:** 116
- **Total carbs:** 7 g
- **Protein:** 4 g
- **Fat:** 8 g
- **Fiber:** 0 g

189. Cinnamon Apple Popcorn

Preparation Time: 10 minutes
Cooking Time: 40 minutes
Servings: 11
Ingredients:

- 4 tbsp. margarine, melted

What you'll need from the store cupboard:

- 10 cup plain popcorn
- 2 cup dried apple rings, unsweetened and chopped
- ½ cup walnuts, chopped
- 2 tbsp. coconut sugar
- 1 tsp. cinnamon
- ½ tsp. vanilla

Directions:
1. Heat oven to 250° F.
2. Place chopped apples in a 9x13-inch baking dish and bake for 20 minutes. Remove from oven and stir in popcorn and nuts.
3. In a small bowl, whisk together margarine, vanilla, coconut sugar, and cinnamon. Drizzle evenly over popcorn and toss to coat.
4. Bake 30 minutes, stirring quickly every 10 minutes. If apples start to turn a dark brown, remove immediately.
5. Pout onto waxed paper to cool for at least 30 minutes. Store in an airtight container. The serving size is 1 cup.

Nutrition:
- **Calories:** 133
- **Total carbs:** 14 g
- **Net carbs:** 11 g
- **Protein:** 3 g
- **Fat:** 8 g
- **Fiber:** 3 g

190. Blackberry Crostata

Preparation Time: 10 minutes
Cooking Time: 40 minutes
Servings: 6
Ingredients:

- 1 9-inch pie crust, unbaked
- 2 cup fresh blackberries
- Juice and zest of 1 lemon
- 2 tbsp. butter, soft

What you'll need from the store cupboard:

- 3 tbsp. maple sugar, divided
- 2 tbsp. cornstarch

Directions:
1. Heat oven to 425° F. Line a large baking sheet with parchment paper and unroll pie crust in pan.
2. In a medium bowl, combine blackberries, 2 tbsp. of maple sugar, lemon juice and zest, and cornstarch. Spoon onto crust leaving a 2-inch edge. Fold and crimp the edges.
3. Dot the berries with 1 tbsp. of butter. Brush the crust edge with remaining butter and sprinkle crust and fruit with remaining maple sugar.
4. Bake for 20 to 22 minutes or until golden brown. Cool before cutting and serving.

Nutrition:
- **Calories:** 206
- **Total carbs:** 24 g
- **Net carbs:** 21 g
- **Protein:** 2 g
- **Fat:** 11 g
- **Fiber:** 3 g

191. Chia and Raspberry Pudding

Preparation Time: 10 minutes
Cooking Time: 0 minutes
Servings: 4
Ingredients:

- 1 cup unsweetened vanilla almond milk
- 2 cups plus ½ cup raspberries, divided
- ¼ cup chia seeds
- 1 ½ tsp. lemon juice
- ½ tsp. lemon zest
- 1 tbsp. honey

Directions:
1. Stir together the almond milk, 2 cups of raspberries, chia seeds, lemon juice, lemon zest, and honey in a small bowl.
2. Transfer the bowl to the fridge to thicken for at least 1 hour, or until a pudding-like texture is achieved.
3. When the pudding is ready, give it a good stir. Scatter with the remaining ½ cup raspberries and serve immediately.

Nutrition:
- **Calories:** 122
- **Carbs:** 17.9 g
- **Protein:** 3.1 g
- **Fat:** 5.2 g
- **Fiber:** 9.0 g
- **Sodium:** 51 mg

192. Palm Trees Holder

Preparation Time: 10 minutes
Cooking Time: 40 minutes
Servings: 2
Ingredients:

- 1 sheet of puff pastry
- ½ cup coconut sugar

Directions:
1. Stretch the puff pastry sheet.
2. Pour the sugar over and fold the puff pastry sheet in half.
3. Put a thin layer of coconut sugar on top and fold the puff pastry in half again.
4. Roll the puff pastry sheet from both ends towards the center (creating the shape of the palm tree).

5. Cut into sheets 5 to 8 mm thick.
6. Preheat the air fryer to 180° C and put the palm trees in the basket.
7. Set the timer for about 10 minutes at 180° C.

Nutrition:
- **Calories:** 108
- **Carbs:** 29 g
- **Protein:** 4 g
- **Fat:** 12 g
- **Cholesterol:** 56 g

193. Almond Cheesecake Bites

Preparation Time: 10 minutes
Cooking Time: 40 minutes
Servings: 6
Ingredients:
- ½ cup reduced-fat cream cheese, soft

What you'll need from the store cupboard:
- ½ cup almonds, ground fine
- ¼ cup almond butter
- 2 drops liquid stevia

Directions:
1. In a large bowl, beat cream cheese, almond butter, and stevia on high speed until the mixture is smooth and creamy. Cover and chill for 30 minutes.
2. Use your hands to shape the mixture into 12 balls.
3. Place the ground almonds on a shallow plate. Roll the balls in the nuts completely covering all sides. Store in an airtight container in the refrigerator.

Nutrition:
- **Calories:** 68
- **Total carbs:** 3 g
- **Net carbs:** 2 g
- **Protein:** 5 g
- **Fat:** 5 g
- **Fiber:** 1 g

194. Strawberry Mousse

Preparation Time: 10 minutes
Cooking Time: 30 minutes
Servings: 6
Ingredients:
- 1 ½ cups fresh strawberries, hulled
- 1 ²/₃ cups chilled unsweetened almond milk
- 2 to 3 drops of liquid stevia
- 1 tsp. organic vanilla extract

Directions:
1. In a food processor, add all the ingredients and pulse until smooth.
2. Transfer into serving bowls and serve.

Meal prep tip: Transfer the mousse into an airtight container. Cover the containers and refrigerate for up to 3 days.

Nutrition:
- **Calories:** 25
- **Total carbs:** 3.4 g
- **Protein:** 0.5 g
- **Total fat:** 1.1g
- **Saturated fat:** 0.1 g
- **Cholesterol:** 0 mg
- **Sugar:** 1.9 g
- **Fiber:** 1 g
- **Sodium:** 50 mg
- **Potassium:** 109 mg

195. Blueberry Lemon "Cup" Cakes

Preparation Time: 10 minutes
Cooking Time: 40 minutes
Servings: 5
Ingredients:

- 4 eggs
- ½ cup coconut milk
- ½ cup blueberries
- 2 tbsp. lemon zest

What you'll need from the store cupboard:

- ½ cup + 1 tsp. coconut flour
- ¼ cup coconut sugar
- ¼ cup coconut oil, melted
- 1 tsp. baking soda
- ½ tsp. lemon extract
- ¼ tsp. stevia extract
- Pinch salt

Directions:

1. In a small bowl, toss berries in the 1 tsp. of flour.
2. In a large bowl, stir together the remaining flour, coconut sugar, baking soda, salt, and zest.
3. Add the remaining ingredients and mix well. Fold in the blueberries.
4. Divide batter evenly into 5 coffee cups. Microwave, one at a time, for 90 seconds, or until they pass the toothpick test.

Nutrition:

- **Calories:** 263
- **Total carbs:** 14 g
- **Net carbs:** 12 g
- **Protein:** 5 g
- **Fat:** 20 g
- **Fiber:** 2 g

196. Baked Maple Custard

Preparation Time: 10 minutes
Cooking Time: 40 minutes
Servings: 6
Ingredients:

- 2 ½ cup half-and-half
- ½ cup egg substitute

What you'll need from the store cupboard:

- 3 cup boiling water
- ¼ cup coconut sugar
- 2 tbsp. sugar-free maple syrup - 2 tsp. vanilla
- Dash nutmeg
- Nonstick cooking spray

Directions:

1. Heat oven to 325° F. Lightly spray 6 custard cups or ramekins with cooking spray.
2. In a large bowl, whisk together half-n-half, egg substitute, coconut sugar, vanilla, and nutmeg. Pour evenly into prepared custard cups. Place cups in a 13x9-inch baking dish.
3. Pour boiling water around, being careful not to splash it into, the cups. Bake 1 hour 15 minutes, centers will not be completely set.
4. Remove cups from the pan and cool completely. Cover and chill overnight.
5. Just before serving, drizzle with the maple syrup.

Nutrition:

- **Calories:** 190
- **Total carbs:** 15 g
- **Protein:** 5 g **Fat:** 12 g
- **Fiber:** 0 g

197. Almond Flour Crackers

Preparation Time: 10 minutes
Cooking Time: 40 minutes
Servings: 8
Ingredients:

- ½ cup coconut oil, melted

What you'll need from the store cupboard:

- 1 ½ cups almond flour
- ¼ cup Stevia

Directions:

1. Heat oven to 350° F. Line a cookie sheet with parchment paper.
2. In a mixing bowl, combine all ingredients and mix well.
3. Spread dough onto prepared cookie sheet, ¼-inch thick. Use a paring knife to score into 24 crackers.
4. Bake 10 to 15 minutes or until golden brown.
5. Separate and store in an airtight container.

Nutrition:

- **Calories:** 281
- **Total carbs:** 16 g
- **Net carbs:** 14 g
- **Protein:** 4 g **Fat:** 23 g
- **Fiber:** 2 g

198. Cream Cheese Pound Cake

Preparation Time: 10 minutes
Cooking Time: 40 minutes
Servings: 14
Ingredients:

- 4 eggs
- 3 ½ oz. cream cheese, soft
- 4 tbsp. butter, soft

What you'll need from the store cupboard:

- 1 ¼ cup almond flour
- ¾ cup coconut sugar
- 1 tsp. baking powder
- 1 tsp. vanilla - ¼ tsp. salt
- Butter flavored cooking spray

Directions:

1. Heat oven to 350° F. Spray an 8-inch loaf pan with cooking spray.
2. In a medium bowl, combine flour, baking powder, and salt. In a large bowl, beat butter and coconut sugar until light and fluffy. And cream cheese and vanilla and beat well. Add the eggs, one at a time, beating after each one. Stir in the dry ingredients until thoroughly combined.
3. Pour into prepared pan and bake 30 to 40 minutes or cake passes the toothpick test. Let cool for 10 minutes in the pan, then invert onto a serving plate. Slice and serve.

Nutrition:

- **Calories:** 202 **Fiber:** 1 g
- **Total carbs:** 15 g
- **Net carbs:** 14 g
- **Protein:** 5 g **Fat:** 13 g

199. Oatmeal Peanut Butter Bars

Preparation Time: 10 minutes
Cooking Time: 40 minutes
Servings: 10
Ingredients:

- ½ cup almond milk, unsweetened

What you'll need from the store cupboard:

- 1 cup oats
- ¼ cup agave syrup
- 6 tbsp. raw peanut butter
- 2 tbsp. peanuts, chopped
- 1 tsp. pure vanilla

Directions:
1. Heat oven to 325° F. Line a cookie sheet with parchment paper.
2. Place all ingredients, except the peanuts, into a food processor. Process until you have a sticky dough. Use your hands to mix in the peanuts.
3. Separate the dough into 10 equal balls on the prepared cookie sheet. Shape into squares or bars. Press the bars flat to ¼-inch thickness.
4. Bake for 8 to 12 minutes, or until the tops are nicely browned. Remove from oven and cool completely. The bars will be soft at first but will stiffen as they cool.

Nutrition:
- **Calories:** 125
- **Total carbs:** 14 g
- **Net carbs:** 12 g
- **Protein:** 4 g **Fat:** 6 g
- **Fiber:** 2 g

200. Peach Custard Tart

Preparation Time: 10 minutes
Cooking Time: 40 minutes
Servings: 8
Ingredients:

- 12 oz. frozen unsweetened peach slices, thaw, and drain
- 2 eggs, separated
- 1 cup skim milk
- 4 tbsp. cold margarine, cut into pieces

What you'll need from the store cupboard:

- 1 cup flour
- 3 tbsp. honey
- 2 to 3 tbsp. cold water
- 1 tsp. vanilla
- ¼ tsp. + ⅛ tsp. salt, divided
- ¼ tsp. nutmeg

Directions:
1. Heat oven to 400° F.
2. In a medium bowl, stir together flour and ¼ tsp. of salt. With a pastry blender, cut in margarine until the mixture resembles coarse crumbs. Stir in cold water, a tbsp. at a time, just until moistened. Shape into a disc.
3. On a lightly floured surface, roll out dough to an 11-inch circle. Place in the bottom of a 9-inch tart pan with a removable bottom. Turn the edge under and pierce the sides and bottom with a fork.
4. In a small bowl, beat 1 egg white with a fork, discard the other or save for another use. Lightly brush crust with egg. Place the tart pan on a baking sheet and bake for 10 minutes. Cool.
5. In a large bowl, whisk together egg yolks, honey, vanilla, nutmeg, and ⅛ tsp. of salt until combined.
6. Pour milk in a glass measuring cup and microwave on high for 1 minute. Do not boil. Whisk

milk into egg mixture until blended.
7. Arrange peaches on the bottom of the crust and pour the egg mixture over the top. Bake for 25 to 30 minutes, or until set. Cool to room temperature. Cover and chill at least 2 hours before serving.

Nutrition:
- **Calories:** 180
- **Total carbs:** 22 g
- **Net carbs:** 21 g
- **Protein:** 5 g
- **Fat:** 7 g
- **Fiber:** 1 g

21-Day Food Plan

Whether you are just jumping on the diabetic train or you are already used to living without your sugars and empty carbs, getting new meal ideas is always beneficial when following a restricting diet. Here is a 21-day meal plan incorporating some of the recipes in this book, to get you started.

Day	Breakfast	Lunch	Dinner	Desserts
1	Bulgur porridge	Peppered broccoli chicken	Buttery cod	Pumpkin spiced almonds
2	Cheesy low-carb omelet	Flank steak beef	Fish and salsa	Flourless chocolate cake
3	Breakfast smoothie	Lime baked salmon	Teriyaki chicken and broccoli	Berry almond parfait
4	Apple & cinnamon pancake	Coconut lime chicken	Garlicky mushrooms	Strawberry shake
5	Buckwheat and grapefruit porridge	Wild rice salad with cranberries and almonds	Turkey coriander dish	Chocolate avocado ice cream
6	Quinoa congee with cauliflower	Crab legs	Roasted vegetable and chicken salad	Avocado mousse
7	Mushroom frittata	Chicken satay	Shrimp & veggies curry	Raspberry peach cobbler
8	Cherry berry bulgur bowl	Sage beef	Bbq pork ribs	Apricot soufflé
9	Tofu and vegetable scramble	Cajun salmon	Crispy buttermilk fried chicken	Mango mousse
10	Apple filled Swedish pancake	Trout and zucchinis	Beef, olives, and tomatoes	Baked maple custard

11	Vegetable frittata	Easy lime lamb cutlets	Baked lemon pepper chicken drumsticks	Oatmeal peanut butter bars
12	Bacon & eggs	Peppered chicken breast with basil	Green beans in the oven	Peach custard tart
13	Summer breakfast parfait	Pork spare ribs	Garlicky Chicken with creamer potatoes	Walnut-fruit cake
14	Granola with fruits	Homemade hamburgers	Sumptuous lamb and pomegranate salad	Strawberry & watermelon pops
15	Quinoa congee with cauliflower	Bbq pork ribs	Chicken satay	Chocolate avocado ice cream
16	Cheesy low-carb omelet	Pork chops with grape sauce	Roasted vegetable and chicken salad	Raspberry peach cobbler
17	Vegetable frittata	Flank steak beef	Fish and salsa	Baked maple custard
18	Mushroom frittata	Trout and zucchinis	Peppered broccoli chicken	Berry almond parfait
19	Granola with fruits	Buttery cod	Roasted pork & apples	Avocado mousse
20	Tofu and vegetable scramble	Beef, olives, and tomatoes	Garlicky Chicken with creamer potatoes	Oatmeal peanut butter bars
21	Buckwheat and grapefruit porridge	Shrimp & veggies curry	Coconut lime chicken	Walnut-fruit cake

Conclusion

I hope that I was able to convince you of a sugar-free diet. Don't worry! Small setbacks are quite normal, as temptation lurks around every corner. As long as you stop filling your fridge with sugar, we've done our job!

Do not make it too difficult for yourself with the meals, make them interesting and varied. It also takes some time (several months for me) to get used to the new style of cooking and not using sugar.

Thank you for choosing this sugar-free cookbook. I am very pleased that you have read my book and that you have placed your trust in my recipes and nutrition tips. I wish you all the best, the necessary staying power, and the best of health!

Made in United States
North Haven, CT
11 January 2022